# Management for Nurses and Health Care Professionals

Edited by

**Jennifer Clark** MSc, RGN, RM, RHV, Cert Ed
Associate Head of Academic Development and Research, School of Nursing and Midwifery, University of Wolverhampton, UK

**Lynn Copcutt** MSc, BEd (Hons), RGN, DipN (Lond), RNT
Pro Vice Chancellor (Quality Assurance) and Dean, Faculty of Education and Health Sciences, University of Wolverhampton, UK

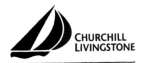

CHURCHILL
LIVINGSTONE

NEW YORK  EDINBURGH  LONDON  MADRID  MELBOURNE  SAN FRANCISCO  TOKYO 1997

CHURCHILL LIVINGSTONE
An imprint of Elsevier Science Limited

© Pearson Professional Limited 2002
© Elsevier Science Limited 2002

First published 1997
Transferred to digital printing 2002
ISBN 0 443 05091 0

British Library Cataloguing in Publication Data
A catalogue record for this book is available from the British Library.

Library of Congress Cataloging in Publication Data
A catalog record for this book is available from the Library of Congress.

The
publisher's
policy is to use
paper manufactured
from sustainable forests

Printed and bound by Antony Rowe Ltd, Eastbourne

**Management for Nurses and Health Care Professionals**

*Dedicated to John Cooper*

For Churchill Livingstone:

Commissioning editor: Ellen Green
Project development editor: Mairi McCubbin
Project manager: Valerie Burgess
Project controller: Derek Robertson
Copy editor: Sukie Hunter
Indexer: Nina Boyd
Design direction: Judith Wright
Sales promotion executive: Hilary Brown

# Contents

# Contributors

**Jennifer Clark** MSc, RGN, RM, RHV, Cert Ed
Associate Head of Academic Development and Research
School of Nursing and Midwifery
University of Wolverhampton,
Walsall

**Collette Clifford** PhD, MSc, DANS, DipN, RGN, OND, RNT
Reader in Health and Nursing Studies
Centre for Health Practice: Research and Development
University of Wolverhampton
Walsall

**Frances Cooper** MPhil, RGN, DipN, Cert Ed, RNT, Dip Health
Studies Research
Director of Nursing and Quality
Royal Wolverhampton Hospitals NHS Trust
Wolverhampton

**Lynn Copcutt** MSC, BEd (Hons), RGN, DipN (Lond), RNT
Pro Vice Chancellor (Quality Assurance) and
Dean, Faculty of Education and Health Sciences,
University of Wolverhampton,
Wolverhampton

**Bob Dredge** MSc, BSc, IPFA
Director of Finance
Royal Wolverhampton Hospitals NHS Trust
Wolverhampton

**Dr Kevin Hogan** PhD, BSc
Principal Lecturer/Head of Department of Psychology
School of Health Sciences
University of Wolverhampton
Wolverhampton

*6 Change in the NHS: strategies and prospects*

**Anne Robotham** MEd, BA, RGN, DipN (Lond), RHV, Cert Ed (FE),
HVT
Principal Lecturer
School of Health Sciences
University of Wolverhampton
Wolverhampton

*3 Managing care in nursing: conflicting philosophies*

**Martin P Yeates** MBA, MIHSM, MHCIMA
Director of Contracts
Royal Wolverhampton Hospitals NHS Trust
Wolverhampton

*4 Purchasers and providers: the 'internal market' explained*

# Preface

There can be little doubt that the outcomes of the reform of the National Health Services (NHS) in the early 1990s in general, and the resulting 'internal market' in particular, are here to stay in some shape or form. With responsibility for deciding which services are to be provided and how they can be afforded having been devolved to local purchasers, and responsibility for the delivery of those services (and any criticism for resulting deficiencies) devolved to local providers, it is unlikely that we will return to a situation where the public can point a finger of blame directly at the Minister of Health. Remember the crisis in the late 1980s about the lack of paediatric ITU beds and qualified nurses?

What better time, therefore, to capture in one book the experiences of academics and practising managers concerning the changes that have taken place? This text brings together in a unique way the knowledge and expertise of academic staff from the School of Health Sciences of the University of Wolverhampton and senior NHS managers who are Executive Directors on the Board of the Royal Wolverhampton Hospitals NHS Trust.

Each author makes a contribution to the running of today's NHS and is concerned with enhancing the quality of service offered to the public. The result is a book which reflects the reality of the management of complex health care delivery systems while enabling the reader to appreciate the way in which management theory underpins practice.

The chapters have been written in such a way that they each can 'stand alone' for the reader who wishes to seek specific information, although the first and second chapters help to 'set the scene' for what follows. Those chapters written by staff of the Trust emphasise current practice (see, for example, Chapter 9) and those written by academic staff from the University, while providing a more theoretical perspective, use examples to illustrate relevance to 'real life' situations and the application of theories to practice.

If you, the reader, have an interest in health service management, either as a student within an educational establishment or as an employee of the NHS, then this text should help to answer some of the questions you may have asked yourself since the NHS reforms began:

- What methods can be used to identify the quality of service provided by health care professionals?
- Why are devolved budgets and the costs associated with clinical procedures now so important?
- When was the Patient's Charter published and what has been its effect?
- How can desirable change be implemented by practitioners in the current environment?
- Where does responsibility for meeting the health care needs of a local population lie?
- Who determines the budget for an NHS Trust?

In answering these, and many other questions, this book should enable the reader to contribute to the operation of the NHS in an informed and more effective way.

1997

L.C.

# Acknowledgements

The editors gratefully acknowledge the contribution made by the following staff of The Royal Wolverhampton Hospitals NHS Trust: Miss Sally Bate, Personnel Manager; Mr Paul Barnett, Personnel Manager; Ms Pam Wakelam, Quality Development Facilitator; Mrs Helen Rowe, Training and Development Manager; Mrs Denise Bott, Deputy Head of Nursing; Mrs Julie Orrillard, Senior Training Advisor.

A very special thank you to Julie Taylor for her invaluable assistance with the preparation of the manuscript, and thanks also to Bev Parker for his help with the graphics.

# Organisations and their management

*Jennifer Clark*

## THE THEORY OF ORGANISATIONS

It is a widely accepted fact that groups of people can achieve more than individuals acting alone. Nowhere is this fact more true than in the health service. Organisations are fundamental to our society; they are essential for the provision of commodities such as houses, motor cars and food. They are essential for the provision of services such as health care, education, information and recreational amenities. The National Health Service is one of the largest organisations in the United Kingdom and many health service employees spend a considerable portion of their lives working within this very complex organisation. If they are to understand how people behave and react within the health service setting they must know more about organisations and the theory that has underpinned our understanding of them.

### Definitions of organisation

Organisations are social arrangements for the controlled performance of collective goals. (Buchanan & Huczynski 1991, p. 95)

The nature of organisations of all types and sizes rests with their shared existence as collections of people working together in a division of labour to achieve a common purpose. As open systems organisations interact with their environment as they transform human and physical resource inputs into product or service outputs. (Schermerhorn et al 1991, p. 31)

Both these definitions reveal three important facts about organisations:

- Firstly they are collections of people who relate to each other because they belong to the same group.
- Secondly they have a common purpose in the achievement of specific tasks or goals.
- Thirdly their performance is controlled to ensure that goals and targets are met and survival of the organisation is assured.

---

**Question 1.1**

What are the specific goals of the organisation or sections of the organisation to which you belong?

---

**Question 1.2**

How does your organisation control the performance of its employees?

---

The study of organisations is not a new activity. The Greeks and Romans were experts in this field and have much to teach us today about how to organise large numbers of people effectively. Handy (1993), however, identified three perspectives through which modern theorists have viewed the study of organisations, namely:

- The individual
- The organisation and its structure
- The systems and interactions within organisations

## Classical theory

The scientific management movement that arose during the first two decades of the 20th century and involved the work of the classical theorists Frederick Taylor, Max Weber and Henri Fayol took a structural approach to organisational analysis. Max Weber (1864–1920) put forward the bureaucratic model of organisational design as the most efficient way to achieving organisational effectiveness. Weber concentrated heavily on the view that workers were innately reluctant to work, were motivated by economic reward, were passive animals that required to be manipulated and controlled into effective employees. This was one view of workers also described by Schein

(1970) as 'rational economic man' (See Box 1.1) and by McGregor (1960) in his assumptions regarding man as an employee, which he labelled Theory X.

Weber's Bureaucratic Model (Weber 1952) relied heavily on a means to an end rationality to create organisational effectiveness. The main principles of his model are described figuratively in Box 1.2. The work of Weber was supported by both Frederick Taylor, an American and Henri Fayol, a Frenchman, both industrialists and with efficiency their prime target they researched successful companies for their major attributes. Their findings mirrored those of Weber, thus adding strength to the scientific management    argument.

## Human relations theory

During the 1920s organisations were growing in size and depending more upon technology. Dissatisfaction was spreading with the

---

**Box 1.1** Assumptions about man – E. Schein (adapted from Pugh & Hickson 1989)

*Rational Economic Man*
Motivated by economic reward man is a passive animal that needs to be manipulated, motivated and controlled by management. This approach underpinned the mass production industry, but broke down when Unions became powerful and jobs became so complex that more was demanded of the employee than automated pairs of hands.

*Social Man*
A social animal who gains a basic sense of identity from relationships with others. The social relationships of the job are all important. Management is effective if it can mobilise and rely on these social relationships.

*Self-Actualising Man*
Man is self-motivating and self controlled. He will be motivated by the job and will integrate his own goals with that of the organisations.
He is adaptive to his environment and has the inherent need to exercise his understanding skills and capabilities in an adult way.

*Complex Man*
Man is variable, he has many motives organised in a hierarchy. These motives change from time to time and from situation to situation.
Human needs fall into many categories and may vary according to the stage of personal development and individual life circumstances.

---

**Box 1.2**   The main principles of Weber's Bureaucratic Model of Organisational Effectiveness (adapted from Mitchell 1985)

*Rules and regulations*
These are essential and are clearly defined to ensure conformity, standardisation and equality of treatment for employees. These are also recorded in writing and open to public scrutiny.

*Well defined job descriptions*
Specific areas of competence should be clearly defined, with all employees aware of the content and boundaries of their role.

*Competence and training*
Emphasis is placed on competence and expertise and training for the specific task.

*Administration separate from production*
White- and blue-collar workers to be kept separate to ensure rationality and objectivity in decision making.

*Hierarchy of authority*
Clear lines of authority are explicit. Communication is vertical. Power and status come with position within the hierarchy.

---

standardised structured approach to work. This dissatisfaction gave rise to the growth of the human relations approach to management. This approach was founded on the early work of Elton Mayo at the Hawthorne Plant in America. Mayo (1975) suggested from his observations of female workers in an electronics factory that the secret of an efficient organisation was to focus upon the individual, her/his reaction to the workplace and involvement in the group. By creating a 'sympathetic' environment for workers the organisation would achieve maximum productivity. This assumption of the individual within the workplace is also described by Schein (1970) as Social Man (see Box 1.1) and by McGregor (1960) in his theory of management entitled Theory Y. The main principles of the human relations theory are described figuratively in Box 1.3.

## Systems theory

The classical theorists emphasise that formal structure and functioning of the organisation is important to efficiency. The human relations

**Box 1.3**  The main principles of the human relations approach to organisational effectiveness (Mayo 1975)

The employee is the key to organisational effectiveness because s/he:
- Views the workplace as a social set second only to home in its importance
- Sets the productivity level, not management
- Considers non-economic awards – e.g. job satisfaction, friendship groups, a pleasant working environment – as valuable as economic awards
- Does not always respond to the work environment alone, but involves groups and subgroups to collaborate and make decisions, thus influencing productivity
- Works more productively in pleasant sympathetic work environments

theorists advocate that the individual and interpersonal relationships are the key to success. The systems theorists, however, throw a different emphasis on to the groups and subgroups within organisations, and insist that it is the inter-relationship and synergy that exists between these groups that is all important.

The premise that underpins systems theory is that the whole is more than the sum of the parts. It is antireductionist in its approach. A reductionist viewing an organisation such as an NHS trust would say that you should look first at the small units, e.g. wards, then at the larger directorates or departments and then at the whole organisation.

A systems analyst would say that you needed to look at the 'whole' by assessing how the subsystems change, work and relate to each other. The systems theorist has a neutral approach to workers, seeing them as adaptive to their environment. This assumption of man is also described by Schein (1970) as Self-Actualising Man (see Box 1.1). The main principles of systems theory are described figuratively in Box 1.4.

## Contingency theory

The basic premise that underlies contingency theory is that effectiveness within organisations is contingent with the right match of internal structure with the external environment. No organisation exists within a vacuum and as the external environment changes so the internal structure and functioning of the organisation must change to ensure its continuing efficiency and survival. Built upon systems

**Box 1.4**  The main principles of systems theory (adapted from Mitchell 1985)

**Systems and subsystems**
All organisations are made up of inter-related parts or elements.

**Holism and synergy**
The whole is greater than the sum of its parts. The total inter-relationship within the organisation is the important factor.

**Open and closed systems**
Systems are open if they exchange information, energy or material with their environment. Open systems have inputs, throughputs and outputs. A hierarchy exists between systems and subsystems.

**Boundaries**
All systems have boundaries. The strength of these boundaries dictates the degree of openness or closure of the system.

**Feedback**
Feedback is vital. Information is fed back to the system regarding its output. Changes are made to the inputs and throughputs to compensate.

theory, effectiveness is seen to be contingent upon the proper match between the external environment and the task, structure, people and technology of the internal environment, as Figure 1.1 demonstrates. When any one of these changes automatic adaptation is required by the other four.

Contingency theory stresses that there is no best way to ensure organisational effectiveness and advocates that managers should conduct a task analysis to determine the approach that best fits their situation. The main principle of contingency theory is described figuratively in Box 1.5.

## The concept of excellence

Over recent years the development of management ideas and theories has escalated, some being far more complex and elaborate than the real world dictates. Some would argue (Torrington et al 1995) that in the world of management theory 'the bubble has burst'. This view, although surprising, has been supported by the work of two American Consultants, Peters and Waterman. Peters & Waterman (1982) studied 43 excellent companies in the United States and from those studies identified eight attributes of the management style of excellent

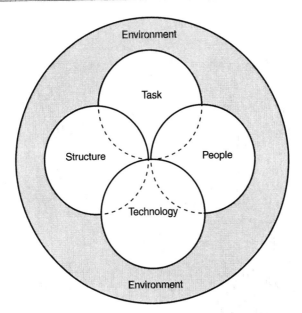

**Fig 1.1**  Contingency theory (adapted from Buchanan & Huczynski 1991)

companies. These are summarised in Box 1.6. This work, although criticised by academics, has been extremely popular and widely read throughout the international business world. The principle that their work demonstrates is one of staggering simplicity, and suggests that the answer to organisational effectiveness lies fundamentally in organisations being 'brilliant at the basics'. In the highly competitive, highly technical and fast-changing environment in which all organisations, including the health service, currently exist, we would do well not to be so concerned with the grand design of the organisation but to return to the basics of management as a job to be done – if it is not, today's delay will become tomorrow's lost opportunity.

---

**Box 1.5**  The main principles of contingency theory

*A best-fit approach*
The right match of the internal environment with the external environment.

*A dynamic approach*
Managers should undertake ongoing task analysis to ensure that the structure, technology, environment and people are always contingent with each other.

**Table 1.1** The major views of the theorists

| The theorist's view of: | Classical theory | Human relations theory | Systems theory | Contingency theory |
|---|---|---|---|---|
| Work/task | Not necessarily designed to be pleasant and to give job satisfaction. | Should be pleasant and enjoyable. Work is an important social set to employees. | Neutral stance. Neither pleasant nor unpleasant. | All aspects must be regularly reviewed to ensure all four are contingent with each other. |
| Organisational structure | Formalised. Clearly defined positions within a hierarchical structure. | Less formalised. Horizontal and vertical lines of communication. Flattened structure. | Clearly defined systems and sub-systems. Hierarchy exists within the systems. | |
| Organisational processes | Legitimate authority. Rules and regulations. Explicit procedures. | Environment of work should be sympathetic to workers. Pleasant surroundings conducive to work. | Functioning and inter-relationships are all-important between systems and between workers and the environment. | |
| People | Pessimistic view. Workers reluctant to work. They require motivation with a system of sanctions and rewards. | Optimistic view. Workers keen to work and achieve. They need to be given the environment in which to excel. | Neutral view. Neither reluctant nor motivated to work. | |

---

**Activity 1.1**

Consider the eight attributes of excellent companies as identified by Peters and Waterman and summarised in Box 1.6.
How many of these are portrayed by your own organisation?

---

**Box 1.6** The attributes of management within excellent companies (Peters & Waterman 1982)

---

*1. Bias for action*
Taking action as opposed to further thinking and analysis.

*2. Customer responsiveness*
Keeping close to the customer and knowing their needs at all times.

*3. Entrepreneurship*
Thinking independently and competitively.
Creating the organisation that can respond to the market quickly.

*4. Productivity through the workforce*
Facilitating employees to participate and share in the success of the organisation.

*5. Hands-on, value driven*
Keeping the whole organisation in touch with the main task of the business.

*6. Sticking to the knitting*
Keeping to the line of business for which the organisation has proven expertise.

*7. Simple structure*
Lean staffing.
Keeping the structure flat with minimum numbers of upper and middle managers.

*8. Flexible climate*
Fostering dedication to the central values of the company while promoting tolerance of individuals who support these values.

## THE STRUCTURE OF ORGANISATIONS

At the start of this chapter organisations were defined as social arrangements which controlled performance to achieve collective goals. One way in which an organisation controls the performance of its employees is through the design or structure of the organisation.

### Definition of structure

Structure is the means for attaining the objectives and goals of the organisation. (Drucker 1974, p. 52)

Formal structures of organisations are typically represented on an organisational chart and stand distinct from the informal or emergent systems with which they coexist. It defines the basic division of labour within the organisation and identifies the number of management levels in the hierarchy of authority. (Schermerhorn et al 1991, p. 309)

Structure includes the allocation of formal responsibilities; the typical organisational chart. It also covers the linking mechanisms between roles, the co-ordinating structures of the organisation if any are needed. (Handy 1993, p. 297)

When designing an organisational structure, a combination of both differentiation and integration is needed. Handy also refers to these two factors but calls them diversity and uniformity. Firstly, any organisational structure must address the need for individuals' jobs to be organised such as to differentiate what the job holder has to do from what everyone else is doing. Secondly, integration is necessary to ensure that by coordinating the activities of individuals the total task of the organisation is undertaken efficiently and satisfactorily.

### Types of structure

#### Entrepreneurial structure (See Fig. 1.2)

Most organisations are not designed but develop and grow with time. Most start as entrepreneurial structures. These structures are small and resemble a web; they have generally developed as the result of one individual having found a niche in the market and not being able any longer to meet the demands of her/his customers on her/his own. Within these structures there is a considerable degree of risk and much depends on personal initiative. Everything tends to depend on the leader, who is the central cog in the wheel. There are few rules and regulations and the organisation functions on the precedent set by the central power source. Size is a problem to the entrepreneurial structure

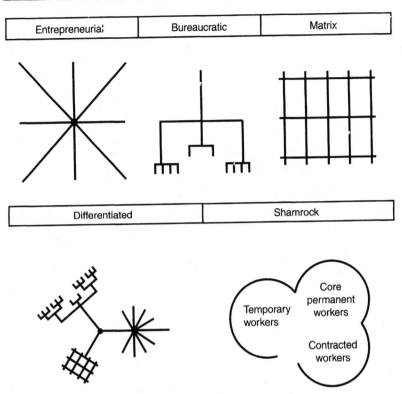

**Fig 1.2** Types of organisational structure: **A.** Entrepreneurial **B.** Bureaucratic **C.** Matrix **D.** Differentiated **E.** Shamrock

and organisations often outgrow the ability for the central power force to control all the activities.

### Bureaucratic structure (See Fig. 1.2)

> Bureaucratic structures are characterised by an advanced degree of specialisation between jobs and departments, by a reliance on formal procedures and paperwork and by extended management hierarchies with clearly marked status distinctions. (Child 1984, p. 7)

The bureaucratic structure is the most common form of organisational structure. It emphasises vertical communication, specialisation and control. Rules and procedures are explicit and well-documented control systems are reinforced by a strong middle management. Power is attached to status and there is an emphasis on routine to create efficiency. The main disadvantage of bureaucratic systems is that they are very slow to react to the external environment because of the

**Table 1.2** Types of bureaucracy

|  | Organic bureaucracy | Mechanistic bureaucracy |
|---|---|---|
| Lines of authority | Decentralised | Centralised |
| Rules and procedures | Few | Many |
| Division of labour | Loose | Precise |
| Managerial techniques | Minimal | Maximum |
| Coordination and control | Informal and personal | Formal and impersonal |

rigidity and centralisation of decision-making power at the top. Burns & Stalker (1961) investigated how bureaucracies could be made to become more flexible and responsive to their environment. They identified two types of bureaucracies – mechanistic and organic. Some more recent theorists refer to organic bureaucracies as 'flattened bureaucracies'. The differences between the two types are identified in Table 1.2.

## Matrix structures (See Fig. 1.2)

In a very rapid and competitive environment entrepreneurial and bureaucratic structures have their obvious disadvantages; this has led to the evolving of the matrix structure. The matrix structure has both horizontal and vertical lines of communication, which allow for a more creative and functional environment. Matrix structures have a flattened hierarchy with top managers holding cross-organisational responsibility, e.g. marketing, finance, quality assurance etc. At operational level project teams exist which are led by personnel with specific expertise for the task in hand. These teams have the power and authority to respond to market needs. This flexibility to the market is essential if organisations are to survive in the current environment of rapid change; however, there is a cost to pay and the disadvantage of this structure is its rather complex communication system. Nurses working within a hospital or community NHS trust that has adopted this structure may find themselves managerially accountable to the director of the directorate within which they work but professionally accountable to the Director of Nursing at Trust board level. This can cause conflicts of interest in some instances. The resource management initiative introduced with the health service in the early 1990s has influenced most NHS trusts to adopt the matrix-style structure.

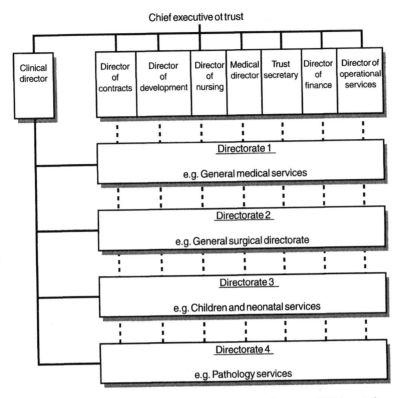

**Fig 1.3** A typical matrix organisational structure as applied to an NHS hospital trust

Figure 1.3 illustrates how a typical matrix-style structure could be applied to a NHS hospital trust.

### Differentiated structures (Fig. 1.2)

It cannot be assumed that the entire organisation will display the same structure. In some larger organisations all three structures may be evident within the same firm. Structures require to be tailor-made to fit the needs of the organisation and the structure that suits the needs of the shop floor may not necessarily meet the needs of the marketing department. A differentiated structure therefore emerges.

What is essential in differentiated structures, however, is that each structure operates autonomously from the others. It is important that the entrepreneurs of the marketing department are free of set procedures and the bureaucrats of the shop floor are free of the power play needed by the entrepreneurs.

**Shamrock structures** (Fig. 1.2)

The shamrock organisational structure can be attributed to the work of Handy (1991). Handy suggests that the current environment of discontinuous change in which organisations exist has resulted in them assuming a 'shamrock-style' structure. The three segments of the structure represent the three types of employee that constitute the workforce. The first segment represents the core workers, who are full time employees of the organisation and are on permanent contracts. Handy emphasises that these core workers are highly paid, few in number and much is demanded of them as they are crucial to the organisation. The second segment represents the temporary workers, who are employed on short-term contracts. A substantial proportion of temporary short-term employees allows an organisation to be flexible and adaptable to the fast-changing needs of the market. To remain flexible in the present climate an organisation must be able to employ staff with specific skills as the work contracts dictate. The third segment represents the contracted workforce; these staff are employed by agencies and ancillary organisations to produce a service or a product required by the organisation. The use of contracted staff provides the organisation with a specific workforce without having to pay the employer overheads incurred by permanent or temporary staff. Handy argues that the shamrock-style structure allows the organisation to be more adaptive to the environment, but offers little security or job enhancement to the employees.

## THE CULTURE OF ORGANISATIONS

As we move towards a new millennium, a transformation is occurring within many organisations. This change, which is evident both in small businesses and in large industries, is also hitting the service industries such as health care and education. At all levels managers are striving for productivity, quality and customer-orientated innovation to replace short-term efficiency measures deemed essential in the past. Management style is changing to facilitation and involvement of staff in the decision-making process, away from the control and top-down management of yesterday. Managers are becoming coaches, team leaders and mentors and in doing so are changing the whole ambience of the workplace. In other words the culture of organisations is changing.

## Definitions of organisational culture

A system of shared beliefs and values that develops within an organisation and guides the behaviour of its members. In the business setting this is often referred to as the corporate culture and just as no two individual personalities are the same, no two organisational cultures are perfectly identical. (Schermerhorn et al 1991, p. 341)

Cultures are created by leaders. (Schein 1985)

A set of values that becomes embodied in an organisational philosophy. (Schein 1985)

Management consultants and academics increasingly believe that a strong cohesive organisational culture has a major impact on the performance and viability of organisations in the modern arena. Schein (1985) identified that a strong culture can both help the organisation adapt to the external environment and achieve integration of the internal environment. This is summarised in Box 1.7.

---

**Box 1.7** Functions of organisational culture — Schein 1985 (adapted from Schermerhorn et al 1991)

---

*Adaptation to the external environment*
Culture can assist by disseminating:

- The basic mission and corporate strategy of the organisation
- Goals and targets to be achieved by the organisation
- Action needed to achieve goals and targets
- Standards and performance indicators needed to measure achievement
- Non-conformance areas and corrective measures necessary to improve performance

*Integration of internal environment*
Culture can assist in the development of a cohesive organisation by:

- Developing a common language for employees
- Determining the criteria for organisational and group membership
- Identifying how power and status is awarded
- Clarifying how rewards and sanctions are earned
- Determining how friendships may be developed and maintained
- Describing how uncontrollable events may be collectively explained

---

## Types of organisational culture

Edgar Schein (1985) and Roger Harrison (1972) have contributed much to our understanding of organisational culture. Schein describes two dominant cultures evident within organisations. He identifies these as Organisation A and Organisation B.

### Organisation A

This is the open organisation with open office space, few closed doors and much dynamic interaction between staff. Management holds the belief that ideas are generated from individuals who are responsible, motivated and committed to the success of the organisation. Argument and disagreement are seen as healthy, safe and positively encouraged within the 'caring family' ethos created by the organisation.

### Organisation B

This is a closed organisation where employees are enclosed within individual offices. The air is hushed and there is little dialogue outside a strict appointment system. Formality and control permeate the atmosphere and deference and obedience to rank is evident whenever the organisation meets collectively. The management holds the belief that ideas and truth come from persons of higher status and experience. People are capable of loyalty and respond to discipline in the carrying out of orders. Relationships are vertical and individuals develop their own niche in the organisation that is guarded rigorously.

---

**Question 1.3**

Which of these two cultures identified by Schein best describes your own organisation and why?

---

You may have had difficulty in deciding which of these two cultures completely relates to your own organisation and you may have come to the conclusion that your organisation's culture is a hybrid of the two. The reason for this is that organisational cultures change: they are dynamic and will be altered by both internal and external influences. For example, a change in leader may be a very strong internal influence on the culture. Likewise a change in government and a subsequent change in political ideology may be a strong external influence on the culture of organisations.

Harrison (1972) identifies four types of organisational culture:

- Power
- Role
- Task
- Person

## Power culture

This is synonymous with entrepreneurial organisations, where the focus is one source of power. There are few rules and regulations and the culture centres on anticipating the wishes of those in power and performing accordingly. Communication is always to and from the central power focus.

## Role culture

This is evident within bureaucracies with hierarchical structures. The organisation is seen as a collection of interlocking roles. Job descriptions are explicit and status and power are awarded to the role performed. Deference to authority is evident and initiative is seen to be counter-productive. Training is encouraged to ensure persons are ably competent to perform their role. Communication is always horizontal and mainly top-down.

## Task culture

This is synonymous with matrix structures. Emphasis within the culture is on expertise and the organisation is orientated towards task and project management. Status for individuals is focused within the task and the proven ability to achieve the goals set. Control is largely invested in the workforce and lines of communication are both horizontal and vertical.

## Person culture

This is synonymous with very small professional organisations, e.g. medical consultant practices, solicitors' offices, barristers' chambers. The focus is centred on meeting the needs of the individual and the organisation is created to meet those needs. Collectivity and the sharing of common aims is evident and communication is usually a process of open sharing. Influence is shared and the powerbase centres on individual expertise. Individuals do what they are good at and are listened to appropriately. This culture is becoming more evident within the modern British family and is displayed within *kibbutzim* and the New-Age traveller communes.

**Activity 1.2**

What kind of organisation do you belong to? Make a list of the set of values and styles of behaviour that characterises it.

What kind of organisation would you like to belong to? Make a second list of the set of values and styles of behaviour you would like to see in your ideal organisation.

Is there dissonance between the two?

# THE POLITICS OF ORGANISATIONS

## Power and leadership

To fully understand the organisation to which you belong it is essential that you understand the internal politics. Politics is about power and influence and using these effectively to achieve identified objectives.

## Definitions of power and influence

An interpersonal relationship where one individual (A) tries to get another individual (B) to do something. This power involves individuals trying to change the behaviour of other individuals. (Mitchell 1985, p. 337)

Influence is the process whereby (A) modifies the attitudes or behaviour of (B). Power is that which enables him to do it. (Handy 1993, p. 118)

Organisations are made up of a mesh of influence patterns and power struggles whereby individuals and groups seek to affect the way others think and behave. Organisations have power as one of their crucial dimensions and it is only by understanding how power is distributed that members can get things done.

Handy (1993), using the work of French and Raven, identifies five sources of power:

- Physical power
- Resource power
- Position power
- Expert power
- Personal power

### Physical power and force

This is the power of a superior force. It is displayed by the bully and is the power of the strong over the weak. With the exception of the police force, prison service and armed forces, physical power is not employed within the majority of work situations. However the dictatorial manager with a very strong physical presence may display elements of this type of power. Physical power uses force or the fear of force to influence and control the action of others.

### Resource power and bargaining

Those who control what others need are in a position of relative power. For this type of power to be effective, the resources held must be desired by others. Resources do not always refer to money. Position, status and information may be equally desired by others and used by individuals to influence the behaviour of others. Resource power uses the element of exchange or bargaining to influence others. Individuals using resource power influence the behaviour of others by offering them obvious advantages for compliance. Recipients must obviously want the advantages for this type of power to be successful and it is often self-limiting in that once the rewards have been achieved behaviour reverts back.

### Position power and procedures

This type of power is associated with role or status. It is often referred to as legitimate power as it surrounds a role and is perceived by others as an attribute of the post-holder just by the nature of the role he or she fulfils. Position power is dependent upon the guarantor of the position reinforcing the power: for example the position power that accompanies the role of Director of Nursing within a trust is only influential if it is underwritten by the chief executive of the trust.

Position power gives managers control over some very important assets – information and access to influential networks of professional relationships could be examples.

Position power invariably uses rules and procedures to influence and alter the behaviour of others; however, ecology may be another source of influence exerted. Individuals do not work in a vacuum and earlier in this chapter we identified that the workplace was a very important social set to individuals. By altering the environment for workers, leaders can manipulate their behaviour. The divide and rule scenario is applicable here: if the manager fears corporate opposition to policies he/she can segregate the workforce. A segregated and disparate workforce adversely affects their means of communication and thus diminishes their corporate power.

### Expert power and persuasion

Expert power is associated with expertise and skill. It is bestowed upon the owner by the recognition of others who respect the credibility achieved by the owner. For that reason it is the least obnoxious form of power as it is always easier to be influenced by someone we respect as being more experienced and skilful. Expert power is never claimed by the owner, only awarded, and it is totally dependent upon the opinions of those over whom it is exercised. Holders of expert power use persuasion as a means of influence. Persuasion is the power of argument and presentation of facts from someone whose credibility is valued.

### Personal power and magnetism

Some people have a charisma of power: by her/his very personality, s/he can influence the way others act and behave. These individuals use magnetism to influence others by invoking a desire to comply with the demands of an individual we respect and admire. Great leaders in history – e.g. Churchill, Napoleon and Hitler – have used this form of power and history has demonstrated that it rises with success and diminishes with failure.

---

**Activity 1.3**

Consider two recent situations where you have influenced the behaviour of others.

Choose one situation from your work situation and one situation from your home or social situation. Analyse which source of power you used and which method of influence you employed.

---

## Power within leadership

Power is not the same as leadership but it is often perceived to be an essential feature of it. It is important at this point to differentiate between power and authority. Power is the strength to exercise control over others, while authority is the power that is accepted as 'legitimate' by subordinates. Rosenbach & Taylor (1993) identify three forms of power in leadership:

- Power over
- Power to
- Power from

### Power over

This is the most familiar form of power within leadership and encompasses explicit or implicit dominance over subordinates. Leaders who rely too heavily on this kind of power to achieve objectives will find in the long term that their relationships with followers are adversely affected and subsequent achievements diminished.

### Power to

This is the power that could be entitled 'empowerment' or power-sharing. This is where the leader releases power to followers by giving them the opportunity to act more freely within agreed guidelines.

### Power from

This is the ability to resist the power of others by ably dismissing their unwanted demands.

## Leadership definitions

A leader is someone who exercises influence over other people. (Buchanan & Huczynski 1991, p. 381)

A special case of interpersonal influence that gets an individual or group to do what the leader wants done. (Schermerhorn et al 1991, p. 461)

Leadership is discovering the route ahead and encouraging and personality permitting, inspiring others to follow. (Stewart 1989, p. 3)

Schermerhorn et al (1991) identify two types of leadership: formal and informal. *Formal leadership* is exercised by those who are appointed to positions of formal authority within organisations, while *informal leadership* is exercised by those persons who become influential within organisations due to their own expertise or control of necessary resources.

## REFLECTIONS ON LEADERSHIP

Since the beginning of time people have sought to understand the phenomenon of leadership. What is it that gives a person this influence over others? Is it something innate within the leader's personality or is it something that can be created and developed? In essence, are leaders born or made – or is neither possible?

**Table 1.3** The most common traits of effective leaders (Handy 1993)

| Intelligence | Initiative | Self-assurance | Helicopter factor |
|---|---|---|---|
| Above average | Independence | Self-confidence | The ability to rise above the particulars of a situation and to perceive it in relationship to the whole |
| Problem solving ability of complex problems | Inventiveness | High self ratings on competence | |
| | Capacity to perceive a need for action and the urge to do it | High aspiration levels | |
| Decision-making ability | | | |

Other frequently cited attributes are: enthusiasm, sociability, integrity, courage, imagination, decisiveness, determination, energy, faith

## Trait theories

Early studies into leadership centred on the premise that the individual was the important consideration and that by identifying the characteristics of successful managers we have the vital clue to leadership effectiveness. This theory was entitled the 'Great Man theory' by Galton (1869). Since Galton there have been innumerable studies into the characteristics of the effective leader but Handy (1993) suggests that the traits summarised in Table 1.3 are common to the findings of most studies.

The common criticism laid at the trait theories of effective leadership was that they did not take cognisance of the situation in which the leader was operating; they implied that an elite corps of managerial talent that was either inherited or acquired was the essential feature. The premise was soon refuted by the style theorists.

---

**Activity 1.4**

Identify a person with whom you have worked and who you rate highly as a leader. List the characteristics that you feel made them so successful.

---

**Activity 1.5**

Identify the characteristics you feel are essential of a Chief Executive of a NHS Trust.

## Style theory

Dissatisfaction with the trait approach to leadership led to a new tactic which focused on leadership behaviour. The leadership behavioural approach, like the trait approach, assumes that the leader is the crucial factor in ensuring effective performance, but instead of concentrating on the innate characteristics of the leader, her/his behaviour or actions are the main target of attention. From the work of the style theorists such as McGregor (1960), Likert (1961), Blake & Mouton (1985) and Vroom & Deci (1970), two dominant styles of leadership emerge: *authoritarian* and *democratic*. The main difference between these two styles is the focus of power. In extreme authoritarianism power rests entirely with the individual – all authority for decision-making, control, reward and punishment rests with the leader – while the democratic leader will share the responsibility for these with individuals or groups. Due to the rather emotive connotations associated with the titles autocrat and democrat, some theorists refer to the *structural* and *supportive* styles of leadership and some refer to those leaders with a 'concern for the task' or 'concern for people'. The findings of the style theorists are best studied in their original work, but Table 1.4 summarises some of the different styles identified by the theorists to give the reader a flavour of their work.

---

**Question 1.4**

What types of leadership style do you witness in your own workplace? Which styles seem to be most effective?

---

**Question 1.5**

Has the recent change in the structure and culture of the NHS affected the leadership style of its managers. If so how?

---

## Contingency theory 'The best fit approach'

The underlying premise of contingency theory is that the leader must be able to diagnose the human and organisational context in which s/he is working to decide which behaviour will 'best fit' the situation. Again, the crucial factor appears still to be the leader and his style of leadership. However, advocates of contingency theory would argue

**Table 1.4** Styles of leadership (adapted from Handy 1993)

| Theorist | Autocratic (Structured leadership) ⟹ | | | Democratic (Supportive/leadership) ⟹ | |
|---|---|---|---|---|---|
| McGregor 1960 | Theory X ⟹ | | | Theory Y | |
| Lippitt & White 1960 | Autocratic ⟹ | | | Democratic ⟶ | Laissez faire |
| Likert 1961 | System 1: Autocratic | System 2: Benevolent autocratic | System 3: Participative | System 4: Democratic | |
| Blake & Mouton 1985 | 1.1 Impoverished management | 9.1 Task management | 1.5 Middle of the road | 1.9 Team management | 9.9 Country Club management |
| Vroom & Deci 1970 | Leader decides | Leader consults | Leader shares | Leader delegates | |

that no one type of behaviour is suitable for every task in every situation. The leader must assess the total situation before selecting the best behavioural style. Fiedler (1967) identified three factors that had implications for the style of leadership needing to be adopted by leaders:

- The extent to which the task is structured
- The leader's position power
- The nature of the relationship between the leader and followers

From this he was able to identify three typical sets of conditions under which the leader may work. Fiedler's work is summarised in Table 1.5.

> The best fit approach maintains that there is no such thing as the right style of leadership, but that the leadership will be most effective when the requirements of the leader, the sub-ordinates and task fit together. (Handy 1993, p. 103)

### Action leadership

John Adair (1983) has pioneered a very effective model of leadership training in Britain, this is known as Action Leadership and is based on the three circles model illustrated in Figure 1.4

Adair identifies three elements that are essential considerations for every leader:

**Table 1.5** Contingency theory (Fiedler 1967)

| Condition 1: Situational context | Condition 2: Situational context | Condition 3: Situational context |
|---|---|---|
| The task is highly structured | The task is unstructured | The task is unstructured |
| The leader's position power is high | The leader's position power is low | The leader's position power is low |
| Subordinates feel their relationship with the leader is good | Subordinates feel their relationship with the leader is moderately good | Subordinates feel their relationship with the leader is poor |
| **Fiedler found** that the most effective leadership style in these situations was: **Task-orientated/ structured leadership** | **Fiedler found** that the most effective leadership style in these situations was: **People-orientated/ supportive leadership** | **Fiedler found** that the most effective leadership style in these situations was: **Task-orientated/ structured leadership** |

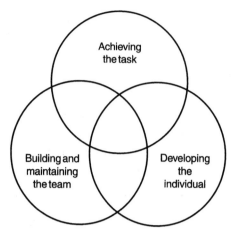

**Fig 1.4** Action-centred leadership: the three-circle model (Adair 1968)

- The needs of the task
- The needs of the individual
- The needs of the team or group

These elements are entwined into each other and should not be viewed separately. Each element affects the other two and there is never a perfect match between them. The skilful manager, however, balances the needs and controls the tensions to achieve optimum performance. He suggests that to do this effectively the manager needs a functional approach that encompasses the roles listed in Box 1.8.

## The new leadership paradigm

### The concept of followership

Over recent years research into effective leadership has shown increasing attention to the follower in the leadership process. Studies of leadership have always assumed the existence of followers, but their roles have largely been seen as passive ones. Recent theories, however, have sought to include the role of followers into our understanding of effective leadership. Within the average organisation there are considerably more followers than leaders. Surely they must have some part to play in the success of their leaders? Until recently all the training and development for leadership has been centred entirely on the identified few, assuming that the large mass of followers has little or no contribution to make. The charismatic and transformational

---

**Box 1.8** Roles of the manager

---

***Defining the task***
Breaking down the task
Determining aims and objectives

***Planning***
Defining options
Setting targets

***Briefing and communication***
− With the team
− With individuals

***Controlling***
Checking the progress of work

***Evaluating***
Assessing consequences
Evaluating individual and team performance

***Motivating***
Inspiring individual motivation
Fostering team spirit

***Organising***
Structuring the task

***Setting an example***
Creating a positive atmosphere

---

theories of leadership are concerned essentially with elevating the goals of the followers so that they have the confidence to go beyond their performance expectations. Lee (1993) identifies some important issues relating to followership: he establishes that everyone is a follower; leaders are also followers in some situations and, as leaders come from the ranks of followers, to become an effective leader one first has to learn how to become an effective follower. Followers are so often classed as subordinates, but effective leadership depends upon followers being viewed as partners, team players and colleagues with a common mission.

**Box 1.9**  The attributes of an effective follower

*Personal integrity*
Loyalty to the organisation and the willingness to act according to their beliefs

*Versatility*
Skilful adaptation to the changing environment

*Ownership of the territory*
They understand the organisation and their contribution to it

*Responsibility for their own career*
They take responsibility for their actions and their own development

Organisations that encourage effective leaders tend also to be ones that foster effective followers. Lee (1993), drawing on the work of Stephen Lundin, identifies the attributes of an effective follower. These are summarised in Box 1.9.

Kelly (1993) stresses that some followers are more effective than others and has developed an instrument to measure follower effectiveness which identifies independent thinking and willingness to question leaders as crucial dimensions (Fig. 1.5).

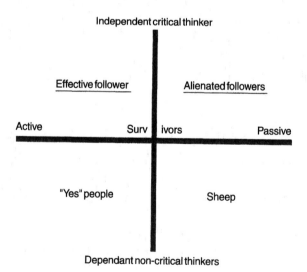

**Fig 1.5**  Follower effectiveness (Kelly 1993)

**Box 1.10**  The leader/follower exchange (adapted from Schermerhorn et al 1991)

| Input by leader | + Effect on follower | = Outcome |
|---|---|---|
| Increased definition/ and direction of a given situation to a follower | Increased esteem and responsiveness to the leader by the follower | Agreed performance maintained |

## Transactional and transformational leadership theory

These theories of leadership are based on the interaction that exists between leader and followers and the ability of the leader to empower followers to act according to and beyond expectations.

### Transactional leadership

This process-orientated approach to leadership encompasses the social exchange perspective. It emphasises that daily exchanges occur between leader and followers that are essential for the maintenance of agreed performance. These exchanges may include increased interpersonal perception and reciprocal influence, as the equation in Box 1.10 exemplifies.

Bass (1989) emphasises that two types of exchange between leaders and followers occur – contingent rewards and management by exception. *Contingent rewards* are specific rewards or advantages that are given to followers in return for meeting mutually agreed performance accomplishments. *Management by exception* mean leaving the follower alone without interference providing agreed performance outcomes are being met.

### Transformational/charismatic leadership theory

Transactional leadership is appropriate for maintaining effective daily performance, but if accomplishment above routine performance is required transformational leadership becomes necessary. Transformational leadership expands and elevates the goals of followers and facilitates them to achieve beyond their expectations. Bass (1989) identifies three facets of transformational leadership:

- The charismatic behaviour of the leader
- The individualised treatment of each follower by the leader
- The intellectual stimulation of each follower by the leader

**Box 1.11** The leader/follower transformation (adapted from Schermerhorn et al 1991)

| Input by leader | + Effect on follower | = Output |
| --- | --- | --- |
| Charismatic behaviour displaying confidence and vision | Broadening and widening of goals and expectations | Performance above expectations achieved |

**The charismatic behaviour of the leader.** This type of behaviour encourages pride in the organisation and respect for and faith in the leadership, and instils a sense of vision in subordinates.

**Individual consideration for each follower.** This emphasises the individual needs of each subordinate and demonstrates a desire for individual development by the delegation of tasks that facilitate learning.

**Intellectual stimulation.** This emphasises the need to encourage and induce creativity in others by facilitating the development of new ideas and by rethinking old practices.

Transformational leadership can be exemplified by the equation given in Box 1.11.

## CONCLUSION

Organisations are crucial to the well-being of the society in which we live: they exist to achieve what individuals cannot achieve on their own. No two organisations are the same; they are dynamic beings, each displaying its own 'personality'. This personality is reflected in the organisation's structure and culture, which may range from hierarchical role-orientated bureaucracies to the flexible task-orientated matrix. To survive, organisations must change with time and in response to the environment in which they exist. Responsibility for the organisation's success in the market-place rests as much with the employees as it does with the leadership. Organisations depend on people to achieve their collective goals and it is the responsibility of the leaders to inspire the workforce to achieve those goals.

## REFERENCES

Adair J 1983 Effective leadership. Gower, London
Blake R, Mouton J 1985 The management grid, III. Gulf Publishing
Buchanan D A, Huczynski A 1991 Organisational behaviour: an introductory text, 2nd edn. Prentice Hall, London
Burns T, Stalker G M 1961 The management of innovation. Tavistock, London
Child J 1984 Organisation – a guide to problems and practice, 2nd edn. Harper & Row, Cambridge.
Drucker P F 1974 New templates for today's organisations. Harvard Business Review January: 45–65
Fiedler F E 1967 A theory of leadership effectiveness. McGraw Hill, London
Galton F 1869 Hereditary genius: an inquiry into its law and consequences. Macmillan, London (paperback edition by Meridan Books, New York, 1962)
Handy C 1991 The age of unreason. Business Books, London
Handy C 1993 Understanding organisations, 4th edn. Penguin, Harmondsworth
Harrison R 1972 How to describe your organisation. Harvard Business Review September
Kelly R 1993 The power of followership. In Rosenbach W, Taylor R (eds) Contemporary issues in leadership. Westview Press, Oxford
Lee C 1993 Followership: the essence of leadership. In Rosenbach W, Taylor R (eds) Contemporary issues in leadership. Westview Press, Oxford
Likert R 1961 New patterns of management. McGraw-Hill, London
Lippitt R, White R 1960 Leader behaviour and member reaction in three social climates. In Cartright D, Zander A (eds) Group dynamics research and theory. Tavistock, London
McGregor D 1960 The human side of enterprise. McGraw-Hill, London
Mayo E 1975 The social problems of industrial civilisation. Routledge & Kegan Paul, London
Mitchell T 1985 People in organisations: an introduction to organisational behaviour. McGraw Hill, London
Peters T J, Waterman R H 1982 In search of excellence. Harper & Row, London
Rosenbach W E, Taylor R L 1993 Contemporary issues in leadership. Westview Press, Oxford
Schein E H 1970 Organisational psychology, 2nd edn. Prentice Hall, New Jersey
Schein E H 1985 Organisational culture and leadership. Jossey- Bass, San Francisco, CA
Schermerhorn J, Hunt J, Osborn R 1991 Managing organisational behaviour, 4th edn. John Wiley & Sons, Chichester
Stewart R 1989 Leading in the NHS – a practical guide. Macmillan, Basingstoke
Torrington D, Weightman J, Johns K 1995 Effective management of people and organisations. Prentice Hall, London
Vroom V, Deci E L 1970 Management and motivation. Penguin, Harmondsworth
Weber M 1952 The essentials of bureaucratic organisation: an ideal type of construction. Glencoe Free Press, Glencoe, IL

# The health services: their macrostructure and microstructure

*Jennifer Clark*

## INTRODUCTION

The National Health Service is one of the biggest and most complex organisations in the world with a budget close to £30 billion and a workforce of approximately 800 000 people. It is also a much loved British institution that is close to the hearts of the British people and is admired and revered by other countries. Despite this however, it has been subjected to criticism and change ever since its inception in 1948.

To lead and manage effectively within any organisation requires an understanding of its history and management structures and this is particularly important within the health service where an understanding of the evolution of the British health-care system will allow contemporary managers to place current developments into context. This chapter will firstly examine the health-care system prior to the emergence of the NHS. This is followed by a review of the philosophy and aims that underpinned its inception. The early experiences of the health service will then be discussed and the structural and financial problems that led to the reorganisations of 1974 and 1982. Finally the chapter will attempt to analyse the effect of Thatcherism on the National Health Service and the ideological shift that has radically transformed the face of health care in the UK by dismantling much of the old bureaucratic structure into a decentralised service which is more self-supporting, competitive and cost-effective.

## HEALTH-CARE PRIOR TO THE NATIONAL HEALTH SERVICE – AN AD HOC SYSTEM

The system of health care in the UK prior to 1948 was a mixture of private and public provision. The private sector provision consisted of private hospitals, general practitioners and voluntary organisations. Public provision was overseen by the Ministry of Health and consisted of local authority hospitals, municipal health services such as sanitation and housing, and community health services such as midwifery, school nursing and child welfare services.

### Voluntary hospitals

These hospitals were endowed by charitable trusts and ranged from large hospitals to small cottage hospitals. They were noted for their high standards of care and their pioneer approach to medicine. Traditionally these hospitals treated patients free of charge, and their sound reputation for high standards of care attracted high-calibre medical staff who would often give their services free of charge in return for the career opportunities offered. Despite being voluntary and supported by charitable monies, these hospitals tended to be selective over the admission of patients, with the very poor often excluded. Many of our large teaching hospitals of today were voluntary hospitals prior to the NHS.

The voluntary hospitals were built and financed by the subscriptions and donations of philanthropists and the altruism of the well-to-do who, in return for their generosity, would be sure of the best available medical care, often given outside hospital, in their own home. This generosity began to wane, however, especially in the 1920s and 1930s, and voluntary hospitals were forced to begin charging for their services. The public responded by taking out private insurance schemes to cover hospital expenses. Funds were always short but despite the financial constraints these hospitals continued to maintain an excellent reputation and provided important care for a substantial proportion of the population.

## Local authority hospitals

The local authorities were responsible for the provision of hospital services to the majority of the population. This was, however, very piecemeal. Traditionally the local authority hospitals had grown out of the Poor Law system, which had provided workhouses for the poor and destitute. Poverty was viewed harshly and potential recipients were made to feel guilty, thus discouraging the poor from seeking help from the state. The workhouses did, however, identify a very high level of illness in the poorer sections of society, which ultimately led to the establishment of local authority infirmaries. These were noted for the practice of subsistence medicine and were often repositories for the chronic sick from the poorer sections of the community. The local authority also provided some hospitals for special needs, e.g. children, the mentally ill, isolation etc. Within the hospital sector, however, there existed a disparity of standards, the hospitals were short of funds and there was a genuine pressure to unify the system.

## The general practitioner service

This was a private service, but the 1911 National Insurance Act introduced by Lloyd George created a health insurance scheme for the working person earning below a certain figure. Contributions were shared between the employee, the employer and the State, and entitled the person to sickness benefit and free treatment by a GP. However, it excluded hospital treatment and treatment for dependants and the unemployed. The scheme was administered by local insurance companies, but it was the precursor to the National Insurance contributory scheme that is fundamental to the health service. Prior to the inception of the National Health Service in 1948, the population had three sources of funding their own health care:

- Private insurance schemes – e.g. friendly societies, commercial insurance companies
- National health insurance
- Self-payment

## Public health services

The local authority was responsible for the provision of public health services. Local Medical Officers accountable to local Health

Committees were established to provide a medley of services including sanitation, water supply, housing and child welfare services.

Criticism of the British health-care system became very apparent between the two World Wars. Two major complaints were made. Firstly the provision of health care was seen to be fragmented with little coordination between the private and public sectors. Secondly, there was inequality in access to health care with little or no provision for the very poor, the unemployed and those vulnerable groups with special needs. More important, however, was the fact that these uncoordinated arrangements were contradictory to the prevailing ideology of post-war Britain, which wanted a comprehensive unified egalitarian service.

As a result of this rising criticism the Government instigated several reports, which included the Royal Commission of 1926, the British Medical Association Report of 1938 and the Beveridge Report of 1942. All pointed to the shortcomings of the service and suggested that services should be unified and made more available to all. The Labour government that legislated the NHS into existence built on the Beveridge Report, which had recommended a universally available comprehensive service free at point of need. Although there was general support for the idea of a universally available health service there was no conformity of view about what form it should take. There were three major pressure groups with varying degrees of power in the bargaining arena:

- The local authorities, who owned hospitals and provided public health services
- The voluntary hospitals, who owned hospitals but required substantial public money to survive
- The doctors, a powerful body whose co-operation was essential as they provided the skills necessary to operate the system

As a consequence of meeting the demands of these groups Aneurin Bevan, then Minister of Health, was forced to abandon his commitment to a unified structure with one administrative body and was effectively forced to create a tripartite system for the administration of the health service. This compromise had far-reaching implications for the newly established National Health Service that came into existence on 5 July 1948.

# THE NATIONAL HEALTH SERVICE (1948–1972) – A COMPREHENSIVE SYSTEM

## Underlying principles

The National Health Service was built on a totally egalitarian premise; this is demonstrated by the following quotes:

> Access to health care was to be determined not by wealth, privilege or advantage, but by need. (Holliday 1992, p. 6d)

> It represented a radical change in the relationship between the individual and the state and it established a firm government commitment to developing and improving the country's system of health care. (Levitt & Wall 1992, p. 10)

> The aim of the health service is to promote the establishment in England and Wales of a comprehensive health service designed to secure improvements in the physical and mental health of the people of England and Wales and the prevention, diagnosis and treatment of illness. (National Health Service Act 1946)

Freedom and choice were fundamental to the new health service. The service was available to everyone and yet individuals were still free to go to doctors outside the service; equally doctors could take private patients as well as practising within the NHS. This freedom and choice did much to reduce the inequalities of health-care provision that had been so obvious prior to 1948. In many respects the National Health Service was a continuation of the health-care provision of the previous 30 years. However, there were three distinguishing changes:

- The service was to be available to everyone regardless of means and was free of charge
- Central government, with the Minister of Health at the helm, was made responsible for the provision of all hospital, specialist and public health services and a tripartite structure was implemented to expedite this provision (Fig. 2.1)
- The cost of the service was to be met by central government. A contribution towards the NHS was levied with National Insurance, but it only amounted to approximately 10% of expenditure, the remaining 90% being drawn from taxation

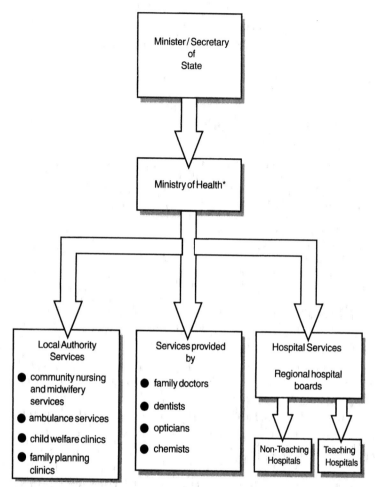

* from 1968, the Department of Health and Social Security

**Fig 2.1**   Structure of the NHS in England 1948

## Tripartite structure (Fig. 2.1)

### Executive councils

These were responsible for the administration of general practitioners, dentists, opticians and pharmacists. The councils included representatives appointed by the Ministry of Health, local professional bodies and local health authorities. The task of these councils was not to provide services but to enter into contracts with members of the professions who would provide services as independent contractors. All members of the population became eligible to register with a general practitioner.

### Local authority services

These were responsible for a variety of public health and environmental services, including midwives, health visitors, community nurses, health education, ambulance services, the care and aftercare of the mentally ill, patients with learning difficulties and the home-help service. The same authorities were also local welfare authorities who provided residential care for the elderly.

### Regional hospital boards

These were responsible for the management of hospitals. 14 regional hospital boards were established which in turn established hospital management committees (HMCs) within their region to control and run their hospitals. Most hospitals management committees had control of a group of hospitals, but some large hospitals and some with specific characteristics had their own HMC.

All 14 regions contained at least one large teaching hospital and within the four London regions there were many more. These teaching hospitals were managed differently by boards of governors appointed by the Minister of Health. Needless to say, they were considered highly privileged by the rest of the hospital service.

## Early problems encountered by the National Health Service

From the beginning the National Health Service was very popular with the public, and by those who had experienced the old system it was acclaimed as a major achievement. Despite this it has throughout its life been subjected to criticism. Initial areas of concern centred mainly on its funding and its structure.

### Funding

The costs of the NHS were grossly underestimated by the planners of the service and the service had hardly begun before concerns were being raised about its cost. The Guilleband Committee was set up to investigate the matter. The report of this committee was unexpectedly favourable and recommended that expenditure on the service was not as excessive as had been previously perceived. It did however point out deficiencies in the system and areas of underfunding that required government attention.

Despite this favourable response from the Guilleband Committee the NHS continued to cause financial concern. There were two main reasons for this: firstly, the service had been established in the belief that the costs of the service would drop as the health of the nation improved. This was proved to be a wrong assumption for many reasons, not least that people's expectations increase with time and familiarity. Researchers have demonstrated that modern health-care costs have risen faster than the rise in national incomes and this has caused a particular problem to the British health service, which is centrally financed. Secondly, there was the issue of accountability of expenditure. The Government determined the amount to be spent on health care and made its decision in the light of other pressing demands on its resources, while on the other hand health authorities, with no responsibility for income, determined a level of expenditure based on need. This inevitably caused a discrepancy between predicted and actual expenditure.

### The tripartite structure

With the passing of time criticism arose over the tripartite structure of the NHS. The major problems were duplication and overlap. The system lacked coordination and it was difficult to provide continuity of care. To the patient, hospital admission might be only one aspect in a total package of care delivered by the General Practitioner, the hospital and community health services, but at grass-roots level it was very difficult to coordinate these three systems that functioned autonomously.

This lack of coordination was made clear by the Government in its first Green Paper on NHS reorganisation, published in 1968 (DHSS 1968). The medical organisations had also identified a wish for a unified service in the 1962 Poritt Report and had recommended the transference of the then local authority responsibilities to newly created Area Health Boards. At the time the Government made no response to this suggestion, but to the medical organisations it became apparent that an official review of the NHS was needed urgently. In the light of the Government's decision to set up a Royal Commission to review the structure of local government, and to appoint the Seebohm Committee to review the organisation of social services, doctors feared that the new rationalised and reorganised local authorities would assume full responsibility for the NHS. Pressure from the worried medical organisations resulted in a review being instigated. This review was originally designed to be private, but in the event it became a very public process and resulted in the publication of the two Green Papers of 1968 and 1970, a Consultative Paper in 1971 and a White Paper in 1972.

In 1972 the DHSS also published a document entitled *Management Arrangements for the Reorganised National Health Service*, also known as the 'Grey Book' (DHSS 1972). The Grey Book set out clearly the Government's proposals for management within the 1974 reorganised National Health Service. The Government advocated a team approach to management, which became known as *consensus* or *diplomatic management*. La Monica & Morgan (1994) define consensus management as: 'No one person or group retaining power; instead decisions are made collectively after discussion of alternatives' (La Monica & Morgan 1994, p. 449).

The Government believed that, by encouraging this team approach to management at all levels within the National Health Service, it would engender more multiprofessional collaboration and co-ordination. However time was to demonstrate that this asset was overshadowed by the lengthy delays that occurred in reaching decisions and in 1974 the National Health Service Reorganisation Act was passed through Parliament.

The basic principle of the reorganisation was integration of the services under new Health Authorities, which incorporated a three-tier structure (Fig. 2.2). 14 Regional Health Authorities (RHAs) were created in England and these were given responsibility for planning, finance and building and the authority to control the 90 new Area Health Authorities (AHAs). Family Practitioner Committees were established to manage primary care (i.e. GPs, dentists, pharmacists and ophthalmic services), and these were accountable to Area Health Authorities. Community Health Councils (CHCs) were also established in an attempt to make health authorities accountable to the public; their powers, however, were and still are only advisory. Some Area Health Authorities were also subdivided into District Management Teams (DMTs).

The structure was a graphic example of the Government's drive towards team management and team accountability, but the very

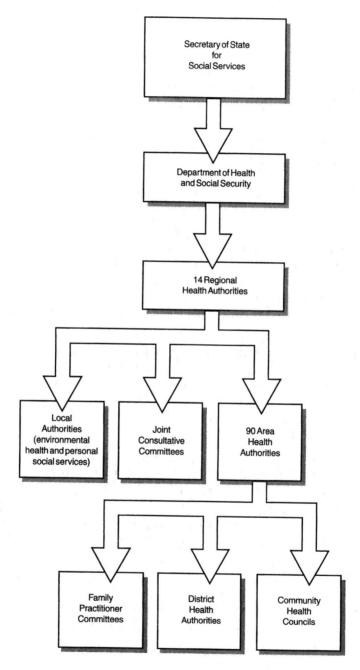

**Fig 2.2** Structure of the NHS in England 1974

bureaucratic multitiered system caused problems from the onset. All levels within the newly reorganised health service believed they should be making strategic decisions and difficulties were encountered between the levels, none feeling that they should be dictated to by the others. This was particularly evident at the middle tier of Area Health Authorities, who often had their financial plans questioned by District Management Teams and Family Practitioner Committees.

A frequent criticism levied against the health service at this time was that it was becoming increasingly more expensive than before, but slower and less effective. The powerful lobby of medical staff continually harangued government for more money at a time when the economy was heavily compromised by the world oil crisis. The government responded by appointing a Royal Commission to examine the NHS. The report, which was published in 1979, submitted findings that were contrary to the widely held assumptions of inefficiency and underfunding in the health service, but it did make recommendations for a simplification of its tiered structure. The new Thatcher government of 1979 adopted some of the recommendations of the Royal Commission, but rejected others, especially those that were expensive to implement, when it published its own consultative document, entitled *Patients First* (DHSS 1979), in December 1979.

## THE ERA OF GENERAL MANAGEMENT: 1983–1989

*Patients First* demonstrated a new Government approach to the National Health Service. Firstly, it was clear from the document that the Government was not prepared to increase spending on the health service until the economy improved. For the first time attention was also drawn to the role played by the private sector in health care and collaboration of the NHS with the independent sector was encouraged. Secondly, it was plain from the document that the Government did not like the top-down centralist approach of the 1974 reorganisation and favoured power at local level, with greater delegation of responsibility to those at the grass roots of care.

The main outcome of the 1982 reorganisation (Fig. 2.3) was the abandonment of the Area tier. Single District AHAs converted to District Health Authorities. District Health Authorities were divided

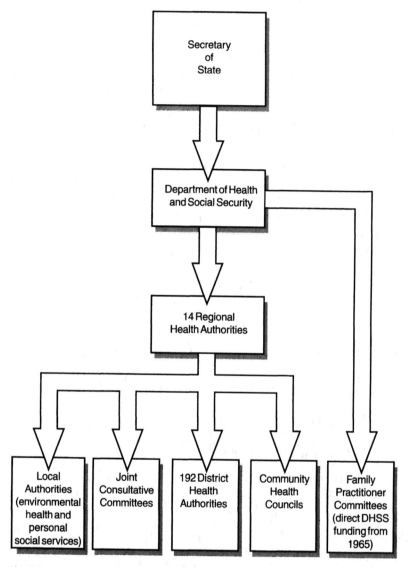

**Fig 2.3** Structure of the NHS in England 1982

into units of management and were encouraged to be less functional and to delegate authority to the units, thus ensuring that decision-making was more local and less remote. Professional planning and the consultative process were simplified to expedite rapid response to local problems and Family Practitioner Committees were reorganised as stand-alone committees with no accountability to the health authorities and financed directly by the Department of Health and Social Security (DHSS).

## Thatcherism and health care

Managerial change was the first political effect of the Thatcher government on the National Health Service. The *Patients First* proposals represented incremental changes to the existing structure and functioning of the health service and it was not until the implementation of general management in 1984 following the Griffiths Enquiry (DHSS 1983) that major change was felt. The report recommended that the health service should embrace the concept of general management, which would replace the old-style consensus management implemented in the 1974 reorganisation. Philip Morgan (La Monica & Morgan 1994), utilising the work of Harrison (1988), used four major headings to summarise the research findings that underpinned the Government's reasoning for the implementation of general management: pluralism, reactiveness, incrementalism and introversion. These are summarised and explained in Box 2.1. The findings of the Griffiths Enquiry reflected Harrison's work in that it identified the following deficiencies within the NHS:

- A lack of strategic drive and vision
- No one person 'accountable' for action
- Delay in decision-making ,
- Professional aims took precedence over organisational aims
- A lack of attention paid to the needs of consumers
- Poor evaluation of performance and little interest in productivity

The Griffiths Enquiry saw the solution to these problems in the appointment of general managers at unit, district and regional level, possibly for a fixed tenure. These managers would be responsible for ensuring efficiency within their organisations and they would do this by ensuring that agreed objectives were met and by the implementation of audit and strategic planning. They would also ensure that doctors became more involved with everyday management issues, that the views of the consumers were sought and gradually incorporated into care and that more accountability was devolved to departmental/unit level.

**Box 2.1**  A summary of the research findings underpinning the Griffiths recommendations (Harrison 1988, adapted from La Monica & Morgan 1994)

*Pluralism*
Within the NHS there was little individual accountability because there were so many players in the policy-making process. Research indicated that managers were not the most influential and the power of the medical lobby was very strong. Decisions were often compromises of conflicting interests and no one person had over-riding authority.

*Reactiveness*
Within the NHS it was apparent that managers were exercising a degree of crisis management, reacting to problems and finding solutions on an ad hoc basis rather than the proactive approach of identifying potential problems before they arose and instigating a preventative strategy.

*Incrementalism*
Within the NHS managers were not taking a radical approach to service provision. They were making adjustments around the edges of existing services and were reluctant to make major changes.

*Introversion*
Within the NHS managers were giving minimal consideration to the views of the consumers. The service reflected more the needs and wishes of the staff.

The Griffiths proposals stimulated considerable debate and criticism, not least from health-care professionals, who viewed them as an attack on professional autonomy. These disputes were handled toughly by the Thatcher government and for nurses the end result was a new management structure that almost entirely abolished the upper echelons of the old nursing hierarchy and had a considerably reduced career structure. At the other end of the NHS structure also, considerable changes resulted from the Griffiths Report. At Government level two new bodies were created: the Supervisory Board (now the NHS Policy Board) and the NHS Management Board (now the NHS Management Executive). 'These two new bodies had the remit to enhance coordination and drive from the top' (Holliday 1992, p. 17).

## THE HEALTH SERVICE SINCE 1989 – THE ERA OF CONSUMERISM

The implementation of the general management initiative marked the beginning of a new era for the National Health Service. This era can effectively be named the era of consumerism. This can be seen reflected in the proposals contained within the two White Papers published by the Government in 1989, *Working for Patients* and *Caring for People* (Department of Health 1989a, b) (Box 2.2).

## THE STRUCTURE OF THE NEW HEALTH SERVICE

### The Department of Health

The main organisational arrangements of the new NHS are shown in Figure 2.4.

*The NHS Policy Board*, which is responsible for the overall policy and strategy of the NHS, is chaired by the Secretary of State. It consists of ministers, civil servants and advisors with special knowledge both of professional and managerial issues.

*The NHS Management Executive* is chaired by the chief executive of the NHS and consists of senior managers who each have a special portfolio – e.g. finance, personnel etc. The Executive has responsibility for the implementation of policy and the everyday management of the NHS.

### NHS Management Executive regional offices

During the 1990s the Government gradually reduced the size and role of the 14 Regional Health Authorities. This was brought about by the establishment of a parallel regional structure under the auspices of the NHS Management Executive. Six NHS Management Executive outposts were set up to deal essentially with the growing number of NHS hospital and community trusts. As trust status became more and more widespread the role of the NHS Management Executive increased at the expense of the Regional Health Authorities, which during 1994 were merged into the NHS Management Executive regional offices. These now total eight in number.

The role and function of the NHS Management Executive regional offices are essentially strategic. Firstly, they are responsible for the

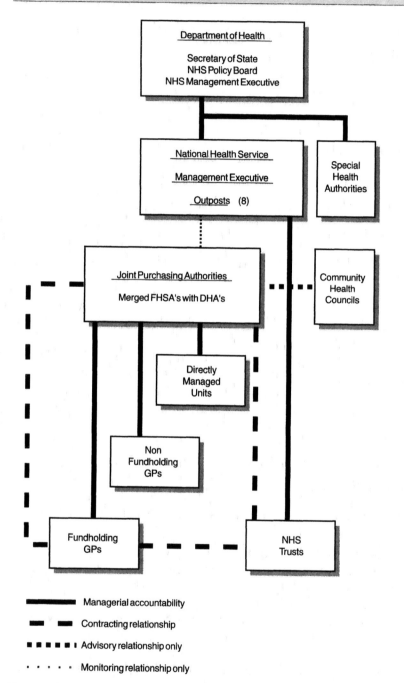

**Fig 2.4**   The National Health Service 1994

**Box 2.2**  The key proposals (Department of Health 1989A)

The White Paper contains seven key measures:

### 1. More delegation of responsibility to local level

To make the service more responsive to patients' needs, responsibilities will be delegated from regions to districts and from districts to hospitals. All hospitals will be given much more control over the running of their own affairs.

### 2. Self-governing hospitals

To encourage a better service to patients, hospitals will be able to apply for a new self-governing status within the NHS hospital trusts. These trusts will be given more freedom to take the decisions which most affect them, such as determining the pay of their own staff and (within limits) borrowing money.

### 3. New funding arrangements

To enable hospitals which best meet patients' needs to get the money to do so, the money required to treat patients will be able to cross administrative boundaries. In future, all NHS hospitals – whether run by health authorities or self-governing – will be free to offer their services to different health authorities and to the private sector. In this way money will go more directly to where the work is done and done best and health authorities will be better able to use their funds to secure a comprehensive range of services.

### 4. Additional consultants

To reduce waiting times and improve the quality of service, 100 new permanent consultant posts will be created over the next 3 years. These will be over and above the already agreed rate of expansion and will also help reduce the long hours worked by some junior doctors.

### 5. GP practice budgets

To help the family doctor improve his service to patients, large GP practices will be able to apply for their own NHS budgets to obtain a defined range of services direct from hospitals. GPs will also be encouraged to offer better services and it will be easier for patients to choose and change their GP.

### 6. Reformed management bodies

To improve the effectiveness of NHS management, regional, district and family practitioner management bodies will be reduced in size and reformed on business lines. They will have executive and non-executive directors. Community Health Councils will continue to act as a channel for consumer views.

### 7. Better audit arrangements

To ensure that all who deliver patient services make best use of resources, quality of service and value for money will be more rigorously audited. Arrangements for 'medical audit' by peer review will be extended throughout the NHS. The Audit Commission will audit the financial accounts of health authorities and other NHS bodies and undertake wide-ranging value for money studies. It will report to Ministers and its reports will be published.

implementation of NHS policy within their geographical boundaries. Secondly, they approve the applications for GP fundholding status and allocate the budget to the fundholding practices. They play a key role in the development of purchasers as they wrestle with the complexities of contracting with providers and they ensure compliance with the regulatory framework for the internal market. See Chapter 4 for more specific details of their role.

## The internal market

### The purchasers of health care

Within the NHS internal market there are two purchasers of health care: Joint Purchasing Health Authorities and GP fundholders.

**Joint Purchasing Health Authorities (JPHAs)** (DHA/FHSA) are responsible for purchasing health care to meet the needs of those living within their geographical boundaries. During the 1990s the number of District Health Authorities decreased, mainly because of DHAs merging to form bigger purchasing agencies. Simultaneously they also worked more closely with FHSAs to corporately purchase health care. This inevitably led in 1995 to the merging of DHAs and FHSAs into Joint Purchasing Health Authorities. The completion date for these mergers is April 1996. The Joint Purchasing Health Authority, whose chairperson is appointed by the Secretary of State, comprises executive members and non-executive members and its remit is to work closely with GPs and other health agencies to draw up purchasing plans and to secure contracts for the provision of that care within the provider units. They also manage the rapidly decreasing number of directly managed units.

**GP fundholders (GPFs)** are in themselves small purchasing authorities. They negotiate and contract with trusts, directly managed units and private health care for services that they require for their patients. Initially, fundholding status was limited to large practices only (those in excess of 11 000 patients), but gradually this criterion has been reduced and some single practices have established consortia with other practices to facilitate fundholding status. Fundholding status has given considerable power and influence to GPs; they always have been the gatekeepers to health care for the population, but the establishment of the internal market has given them even greater authority.

**Non-fundholding GPs.** Some GP practices have for reasons of size or personal preference decided not to become fundholding. These practices remain under the control of the Joint Purchasing Health Authorities. More detail regarding their status and function is provided in Chapter 4.

## The providers of health care

The NHS has two major providers of health care: self-governing trusts and directly managed units.

**Self-governing trusts (SGTs)** are accountable to the Secretary of State through the NHS Management Executive outposts. Each trust is overseen and managed by a trust board, the chairperson of which is appointed by the Secretary of State. The trust board consists of executive and non-executive members. Each SGT has considerable freedom to manage its own work and assets and it does this by negotiating contracts with GP fundholders and Joint Purchasing Health Authorities to provide care that is specific to local needs. Although the SGTs have considerable autonomy they still remain within the NHS and the Government has the right to monitor and if necessary control their activities. SGTs now constitute the largest providers of health care in the UK and it is anticipated that by 1996 95% of hospital and community provision in the UK will be self-governing trusts.

**Directly managed units (DMUs)** are hospital and community units that have not received self-governing status and are directly managed by the Joint Purchasing Health Authority. During recent years, however, they have been given greater powers of management and as more DMUs achieve trust status their numbers are diminishing.

## CONCLUSION

This chapter has traced the development of the health service from its inception in 1948 as the flagship of the welfare state to the 'managed market' of the 1990s. As the health service plans to move into the next millennium it would be natural to predict that its future is likely to be as turbulent as its past. The recent health-care reforms that established the competitive system of purchasers and providers of health care have never been supported by the British public, who took great pride in their free comprehensive service available to all at time of need.

The health service will face many challenges in the future. Some of these will be new challenges as it copes with demographic change and technological advances. It would be safe to predict that the new century will bring medical advances that will push back the boundaries of health care in the UK and, wonderful though these developments will be, they will bring with them ethical, moral and economic dilemmas that are likely to test the very fabric of our health-care system. Escalating costs and the increasing demand for health care from an ageing population is not, however, a new challenge for the National Health Service. Throughout its history, cost has been a fundamental problem underpinning every NHS reorganisation that has taken place; despite this, cost still remains the NHS's biggest problem and is likely to remain so for the foreseeable future. The future is uncertain for the NHS, but 50 years on one thing is certain – we are still trying to get it right!

### REFERENCES

DHSS 1968 The administrative structure of medical and related services in England and Wales (Green Paper). HMSO, London

DHSS 1972 Management arrangements for the reorganised National Health Service (the Grey Book). HMSO, London

DHSS 1979 Patients first: consultative paper on the structure and management of the National Health Service in England and Wales. HMSO, London

DHSS 1983 NHS Management Inquiry (the Griffiths Report). HMSO, London

Department of Health 1989a Working for patients. The health service caring for the 1990s. HMSO, London
Department of Health 1989b Caring for people. HMSO, London
Harrison S 1988 Managing the National Health Service – shifting the frontier. Chapman & Hall, London
Holliday I 1992 The NHS transformed. Baseline Book Co, Manchester
La Monica E & Morgan P 1994 Management in health care. A theoretical and experiential approach. Adaptations for Macmillan edition. Macmillan, Basingstoke
Levitt R & Wall A 1992 The reorganised National Health Service, 4th edn, Chapman & Hall, London
National Health Service Act 1946. HMSO, London

# Managing care in nursing: conflicting philosophies?

*Collette Clifford   Anne Robotham*

## INTRODUCTION

In this chapter a number of issues are explored relating to the impact of changes in health-care management on nursing practice. In doing so it is possible to examine how changing philosophies of nursing care have developed alongside changing philosophies of management in health care. Both hospital and community care are discussed and specific emphasis is placed on community issues in the second half of the chapter.

## ORIGINS OF THE ORGANISATION AND MANAGEMENT OF NURSING WORK

The structures and processes in society at the beginning of the 20th century had a major influence on the evolution of nursing work in the UK (Maggs 1983, Davies 1980, Jolley 1993). These origins are still evident today in the ways in which the nursing profession has reacted to the changing management agenda outlined in earlier chapters.

The beginning of the century was characterised by rapid growth in industrialisation and a clearly defined social structure in which the rules and conventions governing society ensured that every member had a place in the social structure. In that society, the pioneers of organised nursing sought to find a place for nurses that was respectable within the rigid Victorian social order and, at the same time, did not provide a threat to the established medical order. The result of this was the evolution of a hierarchical system of nursing management in which clear lines of responsibility from the most junior to the most senior nurse were identifiable. In this system patterns of nursing work in clinical practice were also hierarchical, reflecting as can be seen below, aspects of life at the turn of the century.

The emphasis on housekeeping skills in early nursing texts indicated the importance for the environment to be 'right' to facilitate the caring role (Pearson & Vaughan 1986). The caring tasks involved creating order in the nursing environment, the wards in the hospital and the home in the community, reflecting the order of the well-run Victorian household. Emphasis was placed on cleanliness and order, a system that served to create a caring setting that was immaculate in presentation. Pictures of hospital wards at the early part of the century, for example, are distinctive for the regimental lining up of hospital beds, the lack of clutter and the polish on all the surfaces.

In the hospital environment the Ward Sister was the absolute authority in the area of nursing care, frequently 'ruling with a rod of iron', while the Matron was the authority in overall charge of nursing. Because of the ongoing association with the voluntary hospitals outlined in Chapter 2 the expectation of patients was commonly of subservience to medical staff and thus by default to nursing staff; and they were expected to comply with whatever treatment was planned for them.

Jolley (1993) suggests that the model of organising and managing nursing was quite acceptable for that time. However, the influence of this way of organising and managing care continued for many years from the inception of the NHS and nurses working in the health service from 1949 through to 1972 were exposed to models of management that had their origins in Victorian Britain. The organisation of nursing work, giving care, could be linked to the models that evolved from the industrial revolution, as seen below.

## Task allocation in nursing care

Hierarchical systems of management were reflected in the clinical areas in the way in which nursing work was organised. Nursing care focused on looking after patients' physical needs and this was divided up into a series of tasks delegated by level of seniority to nursing staff. Thus it was that the junior nurses, for example, were allocated to deal with the 'basic care' needs associated with hygiene while the senior nurses dealt with the more complex procedures such as dressing wounds and drug regimes. Tasks were allocated according to level of seniority, being categorised into a hierarchical domain in which some tasks were seen as holding more status and so fell into the domain of senior nurses. The notion of task allocation in industry was seen as an efficient use of human resources on the basis that workers were trained to optimal performance in developing the skills required in one task. A skilled worker in industry meant increased productivity; a skilled worker in a hospital ward might increase efficiency.

The Ward Sister had managerial control which involved all of the liaison with other departments and communication both upwards and downwards in the nursing and health-care team. Thus, in this system of task allocation, all medical management of care was transmitted to the nurses via the Ward Sister, limiting opportunity for other nurses to develop management skills and reducing the opportunities for multidisciplinary work.

In the early days of the century and eventually in the new NHS, nursing care revolved around the physiological needs of the patients. This reflected the order of the day, for medical knowledge was evolving and largely focused on increasing understanding of anatomy and physiology, disease processes and developing new treatments for the disease.

The focus on physical care has subsequently come under criticism for failing to consider the needs of the whole person, i.e. psychological, social and spiritual needs (Pearson & Vaughan 1986). However, the important point to remember about this model is that when it was established it was reflective of the knowledge level of the day. Moreover, the emphasis on physical care reflected an evolving model of health-care management in which it was acknowledged that nurses were there to assist doctors and doctors were there to heal the sick. Sickness was seen as a physical phenomena as the evolving knowledge base of psychology and sociology did not begin to make an impact on nursing until the late 1960s and early 1970s in the UK. Nursing and medical staff did not focus on physical care because they did not care about other dimensions but rather more because they did not have the broader knowledge base that we have at this end of the 20th century.

This model of organising work by hierarchical management systems, focusing on order in the environment and caring for physical needs by a process of 'task allocation', prevailed without question through the inception of the NHS until the late 1960s and early 1970s. At that point the organisation of the health services came under review, resulting in the first of many changes to impact on health care in subsequent years. This in turn influenced the way in which nurses approached their work.

## CHANGING PHILOSOPHIES: MANAGING CARE IN THE 1970s–1980s

In the previous chapter it was noted that the overall management of the NHS during the 1960s and early 1970s was influenced by a number of organisational reviews. In addition a major review of the ways in which nursing was organised, with the report produced by the Committee on Senior Nursing Staff Structure (Ministry of Health 1966) chaired by Brian Salmon (and so commonly referred to as the 'Salmon Report'). This report was important in identifying weakness in the established order of nursing management in the late 1960s. This included major inconsistencies in style and substance of nursing management, with great disparity in the nature and size of units that Matrons were responsible for managing. Poor delegation on the part of Matrons was noted, with anomalies in the role of Assistant Matron identified.

The Salmon Report made sweeping recommendations involving the separation of policy management from front-line management by creating structures in which 'top management' (Chief Nursing Officers) were responsible for policy, 'middle managers' (Nursing Officers) were responsible for programming the policy and 'first-line managers' (Ward Sisters/Charge Nurses) implemented the policy. This model was adopted and adapted to fit with the reorganisation of the health services in 1974 described in Chapter 2.

One of the key ideas of the Salmon Report was that it would create a structure which enabled the middle managers to stay 'close to patients' while at the same time providing an outlet for career development. In theory this system should have created the opportunity for nurses working at middle management level to develop nursing practice at a local level. The reality was that it very soon became apparent that the inherent hierarchical bureaucracy of health service management was not going to facilitate the ideal of keeping senior nurses 'close to the patient'. With very few exceptions, the Sister/Charge Nurse continued to rule in clinical practice and increasing bureaucracy served to distance the new breed of nurse managers from the bedside. It was within this system, in which task allocation dominated practice for many years, that some nurses started to consider ways in which the organisation of care for patients could be improved.

## Patient allocation

Running parallel with the organisation changes in the health service in the early 1970s, the knowledge base of health care was expanding and understanding of the psychological and social factors that impact on health was increasing. In society at large people were acknowledging the rights of the individual and challenging traditional hierarchies in the social structure. Consequently it was becoming evident to some nurses that a task-dominated, physically oriented system of nursing care was not meeting the needs of patients and clients. Criticisms of using a task-oriented approach to nursing care began to emerge and discussions of fragmentation of care generated by this approach indicated the need to consider the needs of the whole person.

Initially, changes in the organisation of care involved some 'progressive' nursing officers and ward sisters introducing a care management system described as 'patient allocation'. Although this term is widely used now, in the early 1970s it was quite a revolutionary concept as it represented a major break with traditional, hierarchical systems of organising nursing work by task allocation. Patient allocation meant that rather than a nurse being allocated a number of specific tasks to do for many patients s/he was allocated a specific group of patients to care for with the assumption that all tasks for those patients would be catered for by the responsible nurse. In giving this care s/he was not limited to any specific task but would work to meet all the patients' needs within a span of duty.

While this represented a major breakthrough in the organisation of care it had little impact on the overall management of the ward or hospital environment. Although the new approach to care (patient allocation) reduced the mechanistic practices inherent in task allocation, assessment of care needs was confined by the limited knowledge base of nurses at the time. Education programmes still laid emphasis on the 'medical model', i.e. physical needs reflecting the care of the disease process, rather than the whole person with other psychosocial needs also. Moreover, the traditional hierarchy of authority was such that the main liaison between nurses and senior medical staff and other agencies remained at Ward Sister level, indicating a continuation of a task allocation system in some aspects of care management.

Overall, however, the introduction of systems of patient allocation was quite revolutionary as it challenged the established order of task allocation that had operated for many years. The limitation facing Ward Sisters trying to introduce change at this time was that most were working 'in the dark': the processes of implementing change were not widely discussed in health care in the 1970s. Lack of knowledge was also a major contributing factor in the next evolutionary step to develop nursing care – the development associated with the 'nursing process'.

## The nursing process

Following the first tentative moves towards patient allocation as a system of organising nursing work, nurses began to examine what they were doing when they carried out nursing care. Through the 1970s in the UK there was an increasing interest in the ways in which nurses assessed patients' needs and the knowledge required to plan for care, not only physical but also psychological, social and spiritual. This resulted in much discussion about the *processes* involved in care-giving. It was recognised that before giving care this involved *assessment* of needs and defining a *plan* of care to address those needs. Finally it was recognised that if care was to be managed effectively there must be some mechanism of determining the impact of the care, i.e. *evaluating* the care given. These four stages of assessing, planning, giving and evaluating care came to be commonly referred to as the 'nursing process' (Pearson & Vaughan 1986).

The nursing process offered a framework for the organisation of care that nurses, who had for years followed a medical model of care assessment focusing on physical care, could claim to be their own. It was acknowledged that for the nursing process to be properly used there was a need to move away from task systems of allocating work and to encourage wide acceptance of patient allocation systems when managing care. This resulted in recognition that nurses who were committed to patient allocation systems of care management now had opportunity to consider the totality of care provision and challenge the accepted order of traditional working practices.

However, the ideas inherent in the nursing process were introduced into a profession steeped in traditional practices, with the majority only having working experience of systems of task allocation. Little time was given to preparing nursing staff for these new ideas, which proved problematic. Nurses were being advised that they should be 'doing the nursing process' (i.e. assessing, planning, giving and evaluating care) without being given the necessary knowledge base to undertake full physical, psychological and social assessment. It was to take many years before the necessary knowledge base was developed in nursing as a result of changing nursing curricula from a medical model to a nursing model (Clifford 1989). The result was that a government-appointed enquiry was to conclude that the introduction of the nursing process had not been well managed (Department of Health 1987a).

In the resulting confusion for many nurses, the nursing process, a way of describing care, became confused with patient allocation, a system of organising care. This resulted in many nurses stating they were 'doing the nursing process' when in fact what they meant was they were working in a system of patient allocation using a systematic approach to assessing, planning, implementing and evaluating care. It was evident that many of the managers of the day were not conversant with the changes that were being encouraged in nursing and so were not able to provide professional support. Moreover the need to review means of keeping records resulted in many changes of documentation and, as a result, the nursing process became associated with excessive paperwork. However, through the 1970s, the use of patient allocation increased and ward sisters gradually encouraged nurses to take greater responsibility for care-giving and to complete the liaison with the other members of the health-care team. This resulted in a perceived breakdown in ward management. Doctors and other members of the health-care team, who were used to seeing the ward under the strict managerial control of the 'all-knowing' Ward Sister, felt this change keenly, resulting in public debate about the negative aspects of the nursing process with accusations of increasing paperwork at the expense of care (Mitchell 1984).

So it was that the first moves from the nursing profession to identify the focus of nursing care served to confuse rather than enhance the practice of nursing. On reflection, many were working in the dark, for they had no frameworks by which to guide developments in nursing other than traditional models of care based on medicine. However, in the early 1980s this deficit was to be addressed in the form of nursing frameworks or models of care.

## Nursing models

By the 1980s there was general recognition that there was a need for a clear framework on which to base the nursing process. It was from this perspective that nursing frameworks or nursing models were introduced in the UK.

Nursing models provide a way of describing what it is that nurses do. In the USA for many years a number of theorists in nursing had been attempting to unravel the role of the nurse and had began to develop ways in which nursing care could be fully described. This, it was argued, identified the focus of nursing as distinct from medical care. These models serve to illustrate a different way of thinking about patient-care needs from that offered in the traditional medical model, which focused on disease and cure (Pearson & Vaughan 1986).

For example Orem (1980) suggested that nursing was about facilitating the individual to care for her/himself, the so-called *self-care model of nursing*. Nurses who subscribed to this position would carry out the process of nursing with the goal of enabling the individual to care for her/himself. Another approach was presented by Roy (1976), who suggested that nursing was about stress and adaptation. If this view was adopted the role of the nurse was to help the individual adapt to her/his health problems.

Unfortunately, however, many of the early texts dealing with nursing models were complex and unwieldy and those nurses who did attempt to use them often got caught up in the paperwork, again resulting in accusation of excessive paper work and confusion in nursing practice. Although a number of clinical units have adopted

**Box 3.1** The Royal Wolverhampton Hospitals NHS Trust: Ward D1 –
Nursing philosophy

We believe in creating an environment in which we are continually
reassessing our standards of care, methods for delivering that care and
evaluating its effectiveness. The care we provide will be of a holistic
nature ensuring that at all times we respect patients, relatives and friends
as individuals with special needs. We will actively encourage all patients
to attain their maximum potential within the confines of their illness, not
forgetting the special needs of the highly dependent patient and the
terminally ill.

We will endeavour within the ward environment to work as a cohesive
team, striving so that communications are a two-way process, each
individual team member having her/his own professional development
programme. All team members will be actively involved in teaching both
patients, relatives and learner nurses. We will utilise research-based findings
in our clinical practice. The ward team will be encouraged to continually
update their professional knowledge and utilise innovative ideas from all
available sources.

the ideas inherent in authors such as Orem and Roy above, many
others have adopted the simpler idea presented in models by British
authors such as Roper et al (1981), who focus on the 'activities of living',
suggesting that the role of the nurse is to help the patient to fulfil these
activities to an optimal level. Despite the confusion arising out of the
use of prescribed models, one positive benefit of introducing such
ideas was that it promoted nurses to consider their own philosophy
of care and now most wards and clinical units are equipped with some
statement or philosophy of beliefs about the care they are offering the
patients. Such statements are in keeping with the focus on
consumerism in health care today (Box 3.1).

## Primary nursing

With all of these philosophical ideas developing, nurses again needed
to revisit the way in which care was organised and consider ways in
which systems of patient allocation could be extended to reflect the
increasing knowledge base of nursing. From this perspective the idea
of primary nursing was developed.

Primary nursing provides a vehicle from which the nurse can carry
out individualised care of the patient. Primary nursing differs from
the original concept of patient allocation in the late 1960s–1980s as it

is based on complete delegation of care from the Ward Sister to an appropriately qualified nurse. The qualified nurse is responsible for every aspect of care and, because of this, is fully accountable for care given. In the absence of the primary nurse an associate nurse is delegated to carry out the care planned.

Stated benefits of primary nursing for patients/clients included recognition of their 'personal nurse' and associated continuity of care. For nurses, primary nursing is seen as beneficial because it is said to increase personal satisfaction in caring as responsibility is held for the totality of care provision (Ersser & Tutton 1991, Pearson 1988). The concept of primary nursing was again collected from the USA. However, because of differing models of staffing wards and clinical units between the two countries, there was a need to look at ways in which this could be adapted in the UK. In general modifications have evolved around the use of team nursing.

## Team nursing

The ideals of care-giving outlined above were difficult to meet in many clinical situations because of the skill mix of nursing staff working in clinical areas. For example, through the time period of the 1970s to early 1980s hospital ward areas still relied heavily on student nurses to make up the workforce of practitioners. In contrast, nurses in the community worked alone and so had difficulty in monitoring continuity of care in their absence. So, in the UK the concept of team nursing was adopted as a means of modifying some of the ideals of care-giving inherent in patient allocation and primary nursing. This meant that in hospital areas the ward nursing team would consist of student nurses and qualified junior and senior nurses. This model enabled some continuity in allocation of nurses to work with patient groups while at the same time facilitating supervision of student nurses. In the community the existence of a team meant that nurses were able to offer some continuity when they were off duty as named colleagues would carry out the care.

---

**Activity 3.1**

Consider the environment in which you carry out your professional practice. What philosophy of care/practice is evident from the way the service is delivered?

---

**Table 3.1** Developing nursing management and philosophies of care – sequence of events

|  | Nursing care management introduced | Philosophies of care introduced |
|---|---|---|
| 1960s | Patient allocation | |
| 1970s | Team nursing | The nursing process |
| Early 1980s | Team nursing | Nursing models |
| Late 1980s | Primary nursing | |

## Implications of changing models of care

Patient allocation, primary nursing and team nursing changed the balance of hierarchy and power in clinical areas: through the 1980s and into the 1990s the role of the Ward Sister changed radically to become a much more facilitative and supporting role in practice.

These processes indicate a search for identity – a search for something that would distinguish the nursing role from that of colleagues, particularly in medicine. There was no wish to become a separate entity but to undo the shackles of traditional practice in which nursing had evolved as an occupation that, within a hierarchical framework of management, was subservient to medicine, a perception of the role of the nurse that appeared outdated in the world of the 1970s and 1980s.

On reflection it can be seen that nurses approached the changes in the profession in a rather confused and unplanned way. Table 3.1 indicates the sequence of events as they occurred. In effect, at each stage of the process of change nurses were working with insufficient information. It was in the context of this confused professional scenario that general management was introduced into health care.

| **Activity 3.2** |
|---|
| Identify ways in which each of the following philosophies are evident in your own practice: <br><br> • Hierarchical models <br> • Task allocation <br> • Patient allocation <br> • Primary nursing |

## THE IMPACT OF GENERAL MANAGEMENT (1983–1989)

General management was introduced into the NHS as the nursing profession was still struggling to identify the focus of nursing at two levels. The first was the level of care-giving outlined above, where nurses were endeavouring to create systems that would enable them to give individualised care using nursing models/frameworks to assess and plan, implement and evaluate care and systems of care management such as patient allocation with primary nursing or team nursing.

The second level at which nurses were struggling was management, and throughout the 1970s and the early 1980s nurses were seeking to demonstrate capability in management of the NHS. However, many of the nurses in managerial position created by the Salmon recommendations (Ministry of Health 1966) in the 1974 reorganisation of the health service had been placed in their position with little or no training for the role they were to fulfil. Consequently the weaknesses in health service management identified by Griffiths of pluralism, reactiveness, incrementalism and introversion could be identified in nursing (Department of Health 1983).

Strong & Robinson (1990) drew a contrast between the case of doctors and nurses as the NHS moved towards general management. They suggested that doctors were blocking development prior to general management by too much individualism, in contrast to structures created in nursing management which, these authors suggested, resulted in no individualism at all. The same authors noticed that, although the opportunities created by the Salmon review had created a few outstanding leaders in nursing, for others poor management was demonstrated. The key attributes for such failure were seen as hierarchy and ignorance (Strong & Robinson 1990). The reference to hierarchy as an attribute in failing to develop management in nursing showed the negative influence of the established order in the nursing profession. Despite the many organisational changes in the NHS and despite a very changed social environment the power of hierarchical management had survived the decades and at the onset of general management was still serving to inhibit professional development in nursing.

The second attribute contributing toward failed management was ignorance (Strong & Robinson, 1990). Ignorance can be assumed to arise out of lack of appropriate education, an aspect that was given low priority in nursing for many years. Indeed one author reviewing the origins of the nursing profession suggested that the low priority given to education in nursing at the outset could be seen as a compromise in which, at the beginning of the century, the new breed of nurses traded the opportunity for educational development by recognising that societal acceptance would be achieved more rapidly if nursing was to exist in a hierarchical system of deference to medical staff (Maggs 1983). As a result, for a number of years the importance of formal knowledge was not recognised in nursing. Traditionally hierarchical systems of management relied on the power of sapiential knowledge gained by years of service and experience, thus giving 'authority'. Consequently, many of the leaders from the 1974 reorganisation were placed in positions for which they did not have the training. The assumption was that because someone was a good Ward Sister they would make a good Nursing Officer and this attitude pervaded to the top of the profession (Strong & Robinson 1990).

## The advent of Project 2000

By the early 1980s, however, patterns of nurse education were coming under review and it was increasingly recognised that there was a need to provide appropriate skills training for the job at all levels. Although there were obviously many within the profession promoting the need for a radical revision of nurse education to develop clinical care, there were other concerns that ultimately drove this development forward from a management viewpoint, especially a serious concern about a potential shortfall in nursing staff for the future as a result of changing demographic patterns. The result of this review was the implementation of 'Project 2000' as a new way of preparing nurses for the future (UKCC 1986). This was followed by a number of reviews and subsequent recommendations for further educational needs of nursing staff (UKCC 1993). For some this was a positive step to prepare for the new world of management in the 1990s and beyond.

The result of the many poor role models for practice in the era of general management was to leave nursing management in a very weak position to make a major contribution to the development of the new

NHS. It has been noted elsewhere that nurses have not taken full advantages of the managerial changes engendered in general management and undoubtedly this has been a loss to patient care (Dennis 1993). However, given the scenario at the advent of general management, it was hard to see how it could have been otherwise.

The weakness of nursing management in the general management era left uncertainty as to whether the nursing voice would be heard in the new managerial structures arising from *Working for Patients* (Department of Health 1989a). However, as will be seen below, despite initial uncertainties the models that have now been widely adopted include nursing involvement at many levels of management.

As a result of the poor track record many nurses were lost to management roles in the 1980s. Ironically it was at this point that clinical nursing staff who had previously berated managerial systems realised the potential of loss of nursing voice at management level would impact on their capacity to develop nursing in the health-care team. Ultimately the implementation of clinically based directorates, consisting of a team of medical, nursing and business managers to coordinate and manage the activities of clinical units, served to identify the nursing voice in the general management era.

From this shaky start recent indicators are that the nursing voice is being heard more forcibly and positively with the acknowledgement of the importance and effectiveness roles played by nurses in the new NHS trusts. However, in clinical practice the challenges of developing the focus of nursing care remains as the new consumerism model of health care begins to develop.

## THE IMPACT OF THE CHANGES SINCE 1989: CONSUMERISM AND THE NURSING PROFESSION

Clinical units are now generally managed by a directorate consisting of a medical manager, a nursing manager and a business manager. This lays emphasis on multidisciplinary management of care and serves to dilute the previous model of practice in which nurses were both managerial and professionally accountable to a nurse. Within the new system nurses may still be professionally accountable to nurses but managerial accountability may be through other members of the health-care team. This has implications in the wider arena of health-care delivery, as we will see below.

The model of consumerism in the NHS brings with it ideas related to value for money, effectiveness, efficiency and quality of service provision, and consumers' (patients') rights.

---

**Activity 3.3**

How has the recent emphasis on consumerism in the NHS influenced the way in which health-care professionals carry out their day-to-day responsibilities?

---

The notion of 'value for money' was not paramount in the ideologies of the early days of the NHS and so many health professionals are faced with this as a new concept in care-giving, sometimes in conflict with personal ideologies of caring. This, coupled with efficiency and economy in service provision, has resulted in major changes in services with, in some cases, much publicised closure of hospital beds and wards and in some case closure of hospitals. For a profession steeped in historical associations and tradition this has created further managerial challenges. Closures of hospital units, for example, have resulted in the disbanding of teams of health-care professionals who have worked together for many years. This in turn has resulted in a need to build new working relationships, which is an integral part of the change process at a time when there has been little time to adapt to change.

Moreover the changes in health-care services have increased the turnover of patients in hospital, which has made it difficult for nurses to get to know her/his patient in the same way that they did previously. As can be seen later in the chapter, the changes in provision of service have also taken their toll on community care.

Coupled with efficiency, the need to clarify effectiveness in care-giving has infiltrated all levels of service. This has resulted in auditing systems to measure the quality of care provision and the implementation of a research and development strategy to determine the outcomes of care provided (Department of Health 1991a). While most staff acknowledge the need to develop the best quality of care, this intensive monitoring of work activity provides another threat in the changing environment and so may contribute to uncertainties in the unstable workforce of the mid-1990s.

Linked with such initiatives the skill mix of staff has come under review as questions of who provides the most effective care arise. As nursing care provides the largest cost to the health service in terms of hours of work, this is coming under review, alongside the roles of other members of the health-care team. There is an increasing emphasis on multidisciplinary working, which of course serves to challenge the models of nursing care that clinically based nurses have been so focused in developing over more recent years. While few would deny the value of collaborative approaches to health care, placing this on top of the changes already ongoing provides an extra challenge.

---

**Activity 3.4**

If you were tasked with carrying out a review of the nursing grade mix in

- Outpatient departments
- Operating theatres
- High-dependency units

what factors would you consider when determining the number and seniority of nurses required to cover day duty?

---

From the perspective of the key person in health care – the consumer of the service – it is acknowledged that changes in society in which nurses work have changed the relationship between those wanting to use the service and those providing it. Gone is any suggestion of subservience on the part of the patient: the voice of the consumer is paramount. This is strongly evidenced in the Patient's Charter, which states the rights of individual consumers of health care to an effective and efficient health service. Some of the key rights and standards throughout the NHS taken from this charter are illustrated in Box 3.2. The charter has been extended in 1995 and now a number of areas are covered giving specific rights and standards in relation to GP services, hospital services, community services, ambulance services, dental, optical and pharmaceutical services and maternity services (Department of Health 1995).

It is interesting to note that the Patient's Charter has been used to support some of the development of the professional aspects of nursing described above. For example, the right for each patient to have a named nurse, midwife or health visitor to be responsible for

**Box 3.2** Rights and standards throughout the NHS (extract from the Patient's Charter, January 1995)

### Access to service
You have the *right* to:

- receive health care on the basis of clinical need, regardless of the ability to pay
- be registered with a GP and to change your GP easily if you want to
- get emergency medical treatment at any time, through your GP or the emergency ambulance service and hospital accident and emergency department
- be referred to a consultant, acceptable to you, when your GP thinks it necessary, and to be referred for a second opinion if you and your GP agree this is desirable

You can *expect* the NHS to make it easy for everyone to use its services, including children, elderly people or people with physical or mental disabilities.

If your child is admitted to hospital you can *expect* them to be cared for in a children's ward under the supervision of a consultant paediatrician. Exceptionally, when a child has to be admitted to a ward other than a children's ward you can *expect* a named consultant paediatrician to be responsible for advising on their care.

### Personal communication and respect

- You have the *right* to choose whether or not you wish to take part in medical research or medical students' training
- You can *expect* that all the staff you meet will be wearing name badges
- You can *expect* the NHS to respect your privacy, dignity and religious and cultural beliefs at all times and in all places. For example, meals should suit your dietary and religious needs. Staff should ask whether you want to be called by your first or last name and respect your preference

### Providing information
You have the *right* to:

- have any treatment proposed, including any risks involved in that treatment and any alternatives, clearly explained to you before you decide to agree to it
- have access to your health records, and to know that those working for the NHS are under a clear duty to keep their contents confidential

- have any complaint about NHS services – whoever provides them – investigated and to receive a full and prompt reply from the chief executive or general manager
- receive detailed information on local health services. This includes information on the standards of service you can expect, waiting times and on local GP services
- be guaranteed admissions of treatment by a specific date no later than 2 years from the day when your consultant places you on a waiting list

nursing or midwifery care can be seen as a means of ensuring that care-giving programmes are individualised, thus meeting the needs of the patients or client (Department of Health 1995). The named nurse concept arose out of the primary nursing initiative described earlier.

However, many nurses were still struggling to break with traditional practice in developing their models of nursing care at the time when these ideas were incorporated in the Patient's Charter. To implement the named nurse concept required changes in ward management styles which not all clinical areas were ready for. Consequently, while such developments were to be welcomed, the pace of change may have served to undermine the ideology behind setting such standards.

For the practising nurses working within hospital and community units the changes in recent years have taken their toll. Whatever negative views were held in previous years of nursing management (with vast layers of hierarchy, as described by Strong & Robinson 1990) at least nurses did have a line of communication that, in addition to managerial responsibility, was accountable for professional development. The changes in the late 1980s resulted in removing this hierarchy but also resulted in sweeping out many of the 'support mechanisms' available to nurses. Despite the generally negative perception of nursing management, this was a loss when coupled with the other major changes in the health service. The question that remains is how to approach the future in a proactive way in which the experiences for the past can be developed into positive lessons for future development. Before we examine that we shall take a closer look at the provision of community services and the impact of these on staff working in that area.

## The impact on community services

When the NHS became established as the cornerstone of the post- war welfare state (Oakley & Greaves 1995) the 1946 Act allowed for a tripartite structure of management in England and Wales. For community health services this perpetuated the pre-1948 division between community services and hospital services, and local health authorities continued to be responsible for maternity and child welfare clinics, midwifery and health visiting services, vaccination and immunisation and environmental health services. Primary health-care services were divided between the executive councils, who administered family practitioner services, and local health authorities, who administered local personal or community health services. Management of midwifery, home nursing and health visiting services was directly from the superintendent of each discipline via a local discipline-specific nursing officer, and all of these and the services they provided were directly controlled by the Medical Officer of Health (MOH). However, as growth and expansion occurred towards the latter half of the 1960s many local health authorities appointed a chief nursing officer to co-ordinate the three services under the management of the MOH.

For the 1974 NHS management reorganisation community health services was transferred from the relatively democratically appointed local health authorities to 14 regional health authorities who supervised three main structures: local authorities managing environmental health and personal social services; 90 Area Health Authorities with 205 district management teams (in England) who managed hospital and community health services; 90 Family Practitioner Committees who supervised the family practitioner services. However, one of the fundamental differences between the management arrangements for the new 1974-style community health services and the old post-1948 arrangements was the fragmentation of managerial responsibility. Clearly, it brought hospital and community services more closely together but almost completely disintegrated community health services. A Royal Commission on the National Health Service set up in 1979 under the chairmanship of Sir Alec Merrison criticised the 1974 changes, which were said to have too many tiers and too many administrators in all disciplines, to have failed to take quick decisions and to have wasted money. The government of the day set about streamlining the structure, policy-making processes and management of the NHS to ensure that future decisions were taken as close to the point of delivery as possible. In 1983 the Griffiths Report (Department of Health 1983) called for the introduction of new management arrangements to respond to the conclusion that the NHS lacked, at every level of decision-making, a clearly defined general management function. This was to draw together in one person, at different levels of the organisation, the responsibility for planning, implementation and control of performance.

In 1988 the Cumberlege Report was published, which had reviewed community nursing services and made a series of recommendations to strengthen community services and care, followed in 1989 by *Working for Patients*, a White Paper which has underpinned the current market-based reforms.

It is in the light of the Griffiths Report, Cumberlege Report and *Working for Patients* that major changes have occurred within community health-care services, both in their organisation and management, with which this chapter concerns itself.

The influential Griffiths Report showed as its basic premise the weakness of the NHS stemming from a lack of clearly defined management function covering planning and performance appraisal: imprecise objectives, little measurement of health output and infrequent evaluation of performance against agreed clinical, social and economic criteria. Although these general descriptors were identified by Griffiths as applying to the whole NHS system there is little evidence to show that the community services were anything other than a reflection of the whole. It is worthwhile at this stage to comment on management style in the pre-Griffiths era because this also has implications for the way in which subsequent changes were viewed by those professionals working in the community.

## Retaining professional identity

Harrison & Pollitt (1994) make the interesting observation that the pre-Griffiths NHS manager was a diplomat. Rather than shaping and controlling the direction of health services, the diplomat manager helped to organise the facilities and resources for the professionals to get on with their work, and helped to mediate conflicts within the organisation. It was as a result of this style of management – an administrator in many senses of the word – that community health services ran under the direction of the District Medical Officer but with the community nursing services led/supervised by a senior professional for each discipline (e.g. health visiting or district nursing) who acted in this diplomatic role. In many ways this could be a critical reason why there is such a need to retain a professional identity amongst those nursing, midwifery and health-visiting professionals currently working in the community.

Esland (1980) raised the question of whether the professions were using professionalism as 'a strategy for controlling practice' and this became a political ploy in the bargaining process over work definition and independent status in an attempt to protect professional autonomy. Thus it was that, when Griffiths suggested that managers in the NHS should be more concerned about levels of service, quality of product, meeting budgets, cost improvement, productivity, motivating and rewarding staff, research and development, and the long-term viability of the undertaking (Department of Health 1983), there was a sharp intake of the collective professional breath. Where was the professional within this type of structure? Community health care was about professionals working in the community, with people in their homes, and therefore knowing what it was that the community needed.

---

**Activity 3.5**

To what extent is there a need to protect and retain a strong professional identity within a management-led National Health Service?

Are the advantages of so doing going to benefit the patient/client or the professional practitioner the most?

---

One of the key measures within *Working for Patients* (Department of Health 1989a) was that of more delegation to local level to make the service more responsive. This ran alongside another key measure, that of new funding arrangements so that the money was directed to where the work is done best. While the first key measure mentioned had been part of the Griffiths proposals (Department of Health 1983) it had been difficult to implement when unsupported by changes in financial arrangements, compounded by the difficulty of competing with the acute sector for the ever-limited budgets.

In the community, in the period between the inception of the NHS and the 1974 reorganisation, management of budgets was in the hands of the nurse manager, as was the responsibility for day-to-day control of resources. After the 1974 reorganisation the principal aims with regard to nursing were to integrate the hospital and community services and to improve contact and cooperation between nursing and other disciplines at all levels throughout the structure. Managers therefore had to move into teams which were multidisciplinary in nature and led to decision-making by consensus, and clearly this inevitably became a lengthy business. However it is also possible to see that the 'diplomat management' style suggested earlier by Harrison & Pollitt (1994) was most appropriate in consensus management and with its antecedents was the only possible evolution at that time.

## The breadth and depth of community nursing

A result of the many changes in community health-care organisation and management has been to highlight the breadth and depth of services offered and to lead to an attempt to create quality services with efficient management. Nursing in the community embraces a wide range of services provided by district nurses, health visitors, GP-based practice nurses, school nurses, community psychiatric nurses, learning disability nurses, community midwives and specialist nurses such as family planning nurses, Macmillan nurses, stoma and continence nurses. Thus the service ranges from direct nursing through secondary or tertiary care of sick convalescent or very ill people to wide-ranging health promotion and disease prevention over the community as a whole.

The report *Promoting Better Health* (Department of Health 1987b) set the direction for the NHS to transform itself from an 'illness service' into a 'health service', concepts that would require major cognitive changes both within the service and outside it. This prompted GP services to develop more health-promotion-based work and expand disease prevention services, and therefore the FHSAs clearly had to develop their management role. However, prior to this the Government had initiated a review of community nursing chaired by Mrs (now Baroness) Julia Cumberlege, who subsequently reported through *Neighbourhood Nursing – A Focus for Care* (Department of Health 1986) and set the agenda for a complete reorganisation of management of community nurses.

## Cumberlege

The Cumberlege Report (Department of Health 1986), as it was labelled, proposed that the large number of community nurses employed to cover the breadth and depth of community nursing should be organised into what was described as 'core' nursing services and 'peripheral' nursing services. 'Core' services were those provided by the health visitors, district nurses and school nurses and their support staff of enrolled nurses and nursing auxiliaries. 'Peripheral' services were basically all those nurses who worked in the community but were often managed by the acute services from whence they had emerged, and included community midwives, community psychiatric services, community learning disability services and other specialist nurses, including the practice nurses employed by GPs. The Cumberlege review team made a number of criticisms concerning the organisation and management of the existing services, focusing particularly on major areas of concern such as lack of direction and objectiveness of community nursing, lack of team working despite the fact that nurses belonged to primary care teams, and considerable overlap between nursing professionals themselves and other services such as social work.

## Proposals for reorganisation of community nursing services

The Cumberlege Report made a number of specific recommendations, many of which were far-reaching in their vision and have underpinned progressive changes taking place since then.

> Each neighbourhood nursing service should be headed by a manager, chosen for her management skills and leadership qualities, who should be based in the neighbourhood.

This led directly to the appointment of a more able manager, usually with a management qualification, and neighbourhood managers became an important group at the end of the 1980s. In larger authorities they became part of a locality and many health authorities appointed a locality manager who had two or three neighbourhood managers as his/her responsibility.

'Peripheral' nursing groups (see above) were to be responsible for ensuring that their contributions to care were coordinated with the work of the neighbourhood nursing service, under the neighbourhood nurses manager via their own specialist manager.

This, with hindsight, can be seen as a shortcoming of the Cumberlege review team proposals. If all nursing services within the community had been seen as a whole rather than 'core' or 'peripheral', this element of the proposals would not have been necessary.

The creation of a specialist nurse – a nurse practitioner in primary health care – would relieve GPs of many of the tasks allied to diagnosis and treatment of patients.

Cumberlege saw this person as being highly educated, able to take on certain medical protocols agreed with the GP in relation to interviewing and treating patients, providing counselling, support, screening and referral. While in general the nursing profession welcomed this initiative, there was initially disquiet over where this person was to be drawn from, the possibility of medicalising nursing still further and the threat to many possible aspects of the proposed role currently being undertaken by 'core' community nurses and GP practice nurses.

A limited nursing formulary should be approved by Government and the medical and pharmaceutical professions which would allow nurses, specifically district nurses and health visitors, to prescribe directly from a nursing formulary.

It is interesting to note that, despite the agreement in principle from nurses and GPs, it is this aspect of the proposals which has been the slowest to implement, not least because of major concerns expressed by pharmacists on the grounds of prescribing safety and GPs on the grounds of possibly greater drug costs incurred by practices.

The establishment and recognition of primary health-care teams consisting of the medical practice and community nurses which would be controlled and agreed with the relevant health authority. The agreement should also name the doctors and community nurses who are to become part of the team and guarantee them certain rights under the formation and function of the team.

It would appear that while this idea was noteworthy in principle, the balance of team membership on the whole has remained in the traditional medical hierarchical role of doctor/ nurse relationships. The anomalous situation of nurses belonging to a primary health-care team based in general practice and yet managed by a manager in the health authority is one that both parties have difficulty with. Like most structures involving people, much depends on the personalities of the individuals concerned and their flexibility in working practices. Where it works well it does so for the reason of flexibility; where it works badly, the problems are concentrated around suspicion and mistrust, two characteristics stemming from intransigence and often limited recent education.

Presumably as a measure to prevent the above situation, the Cumberlege review report made a suggestion that while the provision of community nursing services should remain under the control of the health authorities, consideration should be given to amalgamating Family Practitioner Committees (the forerunners of the FHSAs) and District Health Authorities.

One aspect of the Cumberlege Report that received post-publication critical discussion was a statement suggesting that overlap of function between various specialist nursing roles could be minimised by breaking down the traditional demarcation lines between health visitors, district nurses and school nurses, with each group using those skills for which they had been educated and yet had seldom used, e.g. health promotion by district nurses and nursing skills by health visitors. Yet at the same time the report highlighted the specialist roles of these groups, and so in essence there was the potential for greater confusion when advocating a generalist approach on the one hand and specialist on the other.

## Models of management of community health-care services

In 1990, as a result of the Cumberlege Report (Department of Health 1986) and the three White Papers *Promoting Better Health* (Department of Health 1987b), *Working for Patients* (Department of Health 1989a) and *Caring for People* (Department of Health 1989b) the NHS Management Executive commissioned a small group of officials from the Policy and Management Executive divisions of the Department of Health and professional groups (plus observers from Wales, Scotland and Northern Ireland), chaired by Catherine McLoughlin and then Sheila Roy, to make recommendations for effective management of community nursing services (North West Thames Regional Health Authority 1990).

After visiting a number of different localities across the purchaser/ provider divide, the group reported on how community services were being managed in a range of organisational models from free-standing community trusts through locality/patch-based services managed by community units to primary health-care teams.

The models proposed by the working groups were seen as appropriate for different sets of circumstances and were to ensure effective management within developing local services, to secure the best possible nursing care in the community within available resources and in a way most suited to the needs of individual users and carers.

The working group set out five different models and briefly outlined the advantages and disadvantages of these as they saw them.

---

**The Community Trust** (stand alone) would manage all community health services and would offer these to GPs, secondary care units, local authorities, voluntary agencies and the independent sector.

---

These would be comprehensive flexible nursing services and the advantage of this model would be to, in effect, retain the status quo because this is where many units would come from and training, monitoring and management of professional staff would be organised by these units. Disadvantages of this model were that GPs might not feel they have full control of their staff and that their own practice nurse might be subsumed into this model.

**Locality management/neighbourhood nursing model**. This is not dissimilar to that outlined above, in that teams of community staff would be managed in localities in either geographical patches or consortia of GP practices or health centres. They would be managed locally under the overall control of the community unit or trust, and GP practice nurses would continue to be employed complementary to other community staff.

The advantage of this model is that it was well known, would ensure continuity of services and community nurses would retain professional support including supervision, advice and monitoring. The disadvantages are that GP practice populations often do not correspond to local authority/neighbourhood boundaries and in addition there may be fewer opportunities for community nurses to widen their traditional roles and cover areas where there have been known gaps, e.g. health visitors working with middle-aged clients.

**Expanded FHSA model** whereby the FHSA would provide community services, acting as a broker for the DHA. The GP would employ practice nurses and contract for other community services from the FHSA.

The advantage of this model would be that the FHSA would have a much greater overview and closer working arrangements with the independent sector, voluntary organisations and local authorities, but the disadvantages are that there would need to be far closer links with the acute sector to integrate service provision and planning with these groups.

**Vertical integration or outreach model**, which could take on a variety of forms: e.g. combined acute/community unit; secondary care unit with community outreach; community unit with acute outreach. Purchasing authorities could contract for complete packages of care, thus leading to seamless care between acute/secondary care unit and community, providing the former was local.

The disadvantage of this model would be that it is illness-focused and that health promotion and disease prevention would be lost.

**Primary health-care team – GP-managed.** This model could be centred on a single practice, a consortium of GPs or a health centre, and the team would include the entire range of specialist nursing services as well as other ancillary services such as speech therapy or chiropody. It would work either by attachment to GPs by specialist nursing staff or direct employment by GPs and the advantage would be a comprehensive team approach relating to a local community.

The disadvantage may well be variations between different practices and limitations within some services, and difficulties experienced by authorities in maintaining an overview of service provision.

## The effect of change on managers and the managed

Probably the most telling effect in the last 5 years of constant reorganisation of community health-care services has been the loss of stability of the management process itself. Senior directors of nursing services have been required to set annual objectives in line with the annual, 5-year and 10-year plans of the trust. This has meant that, where community trusts have been seen to be functioning ineffectively, reorganisation to an alternative model of management has been carried out. Managers with many years of experience in the community have been moved sideways, and have frequently had their focus of control altered, been demoted or otherwise disestablished. A number of managers in the twilight of their working years have taken early retirement or moved to other posts and the result has been a slimmer service with clear vision and developing strategies for community health-care delivery. Managers themselves may not be trained in the same discipline as those professionals whom they manage, but their workforce is very aware that the majority of their managers hold a management qualification, unlike former years when this was not seen as necessary and managers achieved the post by virtue of experience and seniority. The continued difficulty facing managers today is to maintain and create a cost-effective service when policy changes from Government make even greater demands on the service.

The effect on practitioners in the field has been that the professional work force has also been disrupted. Many practitioners, particularly in district nursing and, to a lesser extent, health visiting, have seized opportunities to develop their roles and promote creative approaches to their work. Others in the professional workforce have become very negative and defensive and have found great difficulty in modifying their traditional work practices. Inevitably, where there have been major management reshuffles, nursing and health-care staff have been affected and there is often a period in which the informed observer sees little creative flair in the delivery of health care, particularly in the fields of primary and secondary prevention.

## WHERE TO NOW?

The outline of the developments in community care above gives an overview of the impact of changes in the health service on nursing in the community. It serves to illustrate how a process of change upon change can eventually serve to undermine the ability of nurses to bring a fresh perspective to their work. We can recognise the reaction of staff as described in this study as being a normal response to radical change – particularly a change process that has occurred so rapidly that the ideals of a controlled approach to preparing staff and encouraging participative involvement have not been carried into effect. Overall however, there are few people that would disagree that there was a need for change in the NHS to meet the health-care needs of the 21st century. As health workers adapt to the new models of health care there is a need to consider how nurses can be more proactive in management in the future and build upon the strengths of nurse leadership that are now emerging. The late 1990s are not a time for complacency but a time for action if nurses are to be instrumental in development of management of health care at organisation and practice level into the next century.

---

**Activity 3.6**

As the manager of a group of disillusioned professional staff, what steps could you take to encourage the adoption of a positive approach to change?

---

## Managing the organisation

At organisational level there is a need to ensure that nurses have the appropriate preparation for management to enable them to take a positive and proactive role in the new health services. The need to provide opportunity to address the limitation noted in the Griffiths Report (Department of Health 1983) and subsequently by Strong & Robinson (1990) has been recognised and a wide range of management development programmes are now available. Positive steps have been taken at several levels on this to facilitate the development of existing managers and to prepare the next generation of nursing leaders. As a workforce consisting largely of women, nurses can take advantage of the Government policy to develop managerial potential in women by a programme known as Opportunity 2000 (Adams 1994), or they can avail themselves of an array of programmes designed to develop leadership in nursing (Snell 1995).

## Managing care

The need to break down hierarchical barriers between professional groups is becoming increasingly evident in health care and this in turn impacts on the management of care.

The pace of technological developments, reviews about patterns of work for health-care professionals, the shifting patterns of care from hospital to community, the emphasis on roles of 'carers', ageing populations, economy, efficiency and effectiveness, and so on, have all resulted in questions about skill mix and boundaries of work in the health-care team. In the consumer-driven society the issues that will take us into the 21st century will be to do with maintaining health, maintaining independence and giving choice to the consumer.

From this perspective there is a need to ensure that care services are managed to meet the needs of the consumer. As such, the organisation of health care is coming under review and traditional systems of managing care with prescribed roles for each member of the health-care team are being challenged. The demarcation in roles between health care is eroding and the emphasis on 'patient-focused care' stresses the need to consider the most appropriate person for the care, not necessarily the most appropriate role (Hurst 1995). This process is being enhanced by the recently identified urgent need to review the working hours of junior doctors in the NHS (Department of Health 1991b). Reduction of these hours leads to the question of who will do the work and adds to the erosion of previously clearly identified boundaries of practice between nurse and doctors as nurses take over roles previously held in the medical domain. The nursing profession has responded to this by encouraging the development of roles to meet the needs of patients/clients rather than restricting role development to traditional rules and policies (UKCC 1992).

So for the future the challenge to nurses working at management level and at the front line of care is to contribute positively to the new initiative in health care. Only by making a positive contribution will they be able to influence the direction of health and nursing care in the future (Department of Health 1994).

## CONCLUSION

In this chapter we have examined a number of issues relating to the impact of changes in health-care management on nursing practice. In doing so we have explored changing philosophies of nursing care alongside changing philosophies of management in health care.

It has been suggested that as the radical changes of management began to take hold in the early 1980s, nurses were ill prepared for that role. However, by the mid-1990s there is clear evidence that nurse are beginning to recoup their position and are playing an active role in health-care management for the new NHS. Lessons from the past have indicated that it is all too easy to separate nursing management from nursing care givers in developing different philosophies of care. It is evident now that the multidisciplinary perspective is contributing towards health-care development at a strategic level. It is important that all nurses grasp the ideas inherent in this – multidisciplinary work is here to stay and is being positively encouraged through the NHS. Nurses need to consider the implications of this for their care so that they may be able to define the nursing contribution to care in the new NHS.

REFERENCES

Adams J 1994 Opportunity 2000. Nursing Times 9: 31–32
Clifford C 1989 An experience of transition from a medical model to a nursing model in nurse education. Nurse Education Today 9: 413–418
Davies C (ed) 1980 Rewriting nursing history. Croom Helm, London
Dennis J 1993 How does it feel? In Spurgeon P (ed) The new face of the NHS, Longman, Harlow
Department of Health 1983 NHS management enquiry (Chair R Griffiths). HMSO, London
Department of Health 1986 Neighbourhood nursing – a focus for care. Report of the Community Nursing Review. HMSO, London

Department of Health 1987a Promoting better health – the Government's programme for improving primary health care. HMSO, London

Department of Health 1987b Report on the nursing process. Evaluation Nursing Group, Nursing Education Research Unit, Kings College, London. HMSO, London

Department of Health 1989a Working for patients. HMSO, London

Department of Health 1989b Caring for people. HMSO, London

Department of Health 1991a A strategy for research in the NHS. HMSO, London

Department of Health 1991b A new deal. HMSO, London

Department of Health 1994 The challenges for nursing and midwifery. HMSO, London

Department of Health 1995 The Patient's Charter and you. HMSO, London

Ersser S, Tutton E (ed) 1991 Primary nursing in perspective. Scutari Press, London

Esland, G. 1980 Professions and professionalism. In Esland G, Salaman G (ed) The politics of work and occupations. Free Press, New York

Harrison S, Pollitt C 1994 Controlling health professionals – the future of work and organisations in the NHS. Open University Press, Buckingham

Hurst K 1995 Progress with patient-focused care in the United Kingdom. NHS Executive, Department of Health, London

Jolley M 1993 Out of the past. In Jolley M, Brykczynska G Nursing; its hidden agendas. Edward Arnold, Sevenoaks, ch 1

Maggs C 1983 The origins of general nursing. Croom Helm, London

Ministry of Health, Scottish Home and Health Department 1966 Report of the Committee of Senior Nursing Staff Structure (Chair B Salmon). HMSO, London

Mitchell J R A 1984 Is nursing any business of doctors? A simple guide to the nursing process. British Medical Journal 288: 218–219

North West Thames Regional Health Authority 1990 Nursing in the community. Report of the Working Group. North West Thames Regional Health Authority, Kingston-upon-Thames

Oakley P, Greaves C 1995 Setting the framework – restructuring the organisation. Health Services Journal, 26 January: 24–26

Oakley P, Greaves E 1995 A catalyst for change. Health Service Journal 105: 30–31

Orem D 1980 Nursing – concepts and principles, 2nd edn. Little, Brown, Boston.

Pearson A 1988 Primary nursing. Croom Helm, London

Pearson A, Vaughan B 1986 Nursing models for practice. Heinemann, London

Roper N, Logan W, Tierney A 1981 The elements of nursing. Churchill Livingstone, Edinburgh

Roy C 1976 Introduction to nursing: an adaptation model. Prentice Hall, Englewood Cliffs, NJ

Snell J 1995 Pushing forward. Nursing Times 91(39): 29–30

Strong P, Robinson J 1990 The NHS under new management. Open University Press, Milton Keynes

UKCC 1986 Project 2000 – a new preparation for practice. HMSO, London

UKCC 1992 The scope of professional practice. HMSO, London

UKCC 1994 The future of professional practice – the Council's standards for education and practice following registration. HMSO, London

# Purchasers and providers: the 'internal market' explained

*M. P. Yeates*

**4**

## PURCHASERS AND PROVIDERS

In this chapter, consideration is given to the health service reforms, the reasons behind them and the roles of the 'power players' in the internal market. At the same time emphasis will be placed upon the practical outcome of applying marketing principles and concepts to the National Health Service (NHS). A detailed description of the health service reforms are given in Chapter 2; the following paragraphs simply serve as a reminder to readers of the main issues and to set the purchaser/provider scenario into context.

### Pre-1990

Prior to the reforms, there was a relatively straightforward and bureaucratic delivery of health services. The chain of line management which commenced with the Secretary of State could be traced relatively easily through Regional Health Authorities and Districts into hospitals and community units.

In broad terms, policy was developed and delivered through one chain of command. The recipients of the services, the patients and General Practitioners, were most definitely the 'poor relations' in the service. With the exception of pressure groups such as the Local Medical Committee and the Community Health Council, both with limited power, the recipients of the service had difficulty in engineering change.

In the immediate years prior to 1990, the Government was subjected to increasing and sustained pressure from the media and from unexpected pressure groups, notably the British Medical Association (BMA), in relation to the underfunding of the NHS. Due to the direct management line to Government the criticism could not be deflected, whether or not it was reasonable.

The Government was also, at that time, of the view that the NHS was mismanaged. Investigation by Sir Roy Griffiths had caused considerable concern, and implementation of his recommendations bringing about general management had only slightly improved this perception. Finally, a view was held that the 'bottomless pit' of the NHS, swallowing increasing resources and still arguing underfunding, could not be perpetuated. In the light of these and other factors the Prime Minister, Margaret Thatcher, announced a fundamental review of the financing, management and delivery of the health services.

The review was far reaching and a number of alternative strategies were considered:

- Funding from central taxation
- Funding from an 'earmarked' health service tax (direct or indirect)
- Funding through 'earmarked' National Health Insurance
- Funding the individual citizen through vouchers
- The role of tax incentives and credits
- Various options of 'private/public mix'

With regard to the delivery and management of health services a number of alternatives were also considered:

- Public provision as then through regions and districts (status quo)
- Public provision in the absence of regions
- Public provision through regional strategic planning and management with diminished roles for districts
- Health Maintenance Organisations (HMOs)
- Changed demarcation between hospital and community health services and Family Practitioner Services
- Various forms and ratios of public/private mix
- Introduction of an internal market

The Minister of Health, Kenneth Clarke, introduced the outcome of the review in February 1990 with the publication of the document *Working for Patients* (Department of Health 1989). This was rapidly followed by nine and eventually 11 working papers. The working papers were changed very little following public consultation and the outcome of the review became statute in the National Health Service and Community Care Act 1990.

The working papers were extensive and covered such topics as:

- Health authorities
- Self-governing hospitals
- GP prescribing
- GP fundholding
- Capital charges
- Contracts
- Consultant contracts
- Medical audit
- Training

## District Health Authorities (DHAs) and Family Health Service Authorities (FHSAs) as Purchasers

Following the reforms the Purchaser received a clear and unambiguous role. The requirement was to assess and improve the health status of their resident population by placing contracts with whichever provider was most likely to deliver services to meet their requirements. With effect from 1 April 1995, the majority of FHSA/DHAs aligned (the merger to be formalised on 1 April 1996), providing the organisation with a formal role of payment and monitoring of local General Practitioners, previously undertaken by the separate FHSAs.

One of the most critical changes to the District Health Authority was the membership of the board. Prior to the reforms, the DHA consisted of some 30 members, elected from organisations such as the local authority, hospital consultants and pressure groups. They were politically influenced organisations with, some would argue, a lack of clarity and objectivity.

The reformed organisations consist of a chairman and five non-executive directors (e.g. local individuals involved within the community) appointed by the NHS Management Executive Regional Office, and five executive directors, including the chief executive. The latter group are full time NHS employees, while the former are part time, spending around 20–30 days per annum fulfilling their non-executive role.

## The process of purchasing

The Director of Public Health assesses the health status of the district's population and agrees priorities for investment or disinvestment of purchaser's budgets. In the latter case this may now include certain clinical procedures that will not be purchased, for example, removal of tattoos.

---

**Question 4.1**

Are there ethical dilemmas surrounding the decision of purchasers not to place contracts for certain clinical procedures such as tattoo removal?
   Can you list any other procedures which could be placed in the 'non-fundable' category?

---

The Director of Finance, upon receipt of the purchasing budget, will ensure that the maximum number of priorities are financed within the available resources. When resources cannot support demand, then the purchaser – the Joint Purchasing Health Authority (DHA/FHSA) – has hard choices to make regarding the provision of health care for the resident population.

The Director of Contracts negotiates and places contracts with providers (see below for a definition of a provider) that maximise quality, activity and value for money. Increasingly, purchasers are now, through this process, tendering entire clinical services to providers, with an expectation of maximising economies of scale and obtaining value for money.

---

**Question 4.2**

Are clinical services linked to contracts? If so, what would happen, for example, to the rheumatology service if the Trust loses the rheumatology contract to a neighbouring competing trust?

---

## GP fundholders (GPFH)

Whether one believes that GP fundholders are a good or bad development, allocating resources to GPs with which they can purchase health care for their patients has been the most influential factor in ensuring successful implementation of the NHS reforms.

The general practitioner could, like District Health Authorities, purchase health provision from any provider. The GPs taking fundholding status in the first few years did so in order to change things, i.e. they volunteered, knowing that the decisions they made would have a major influence on local hospitals and the senior medical staff within them. The result was improved waiting times for their patients, improved communications between the practice and the providers of services and improved facilities and services within the practice. It is significant that there were varying responses from providers to the scheme, resulting in some successful providers and some failures, as purchasers decided where they would send their patients for treatment. This led to a significant shift in the NHS power base, whereby consultants working in provider units (e.g. trusts) needed to ensure that they attracted GP/DHA 'business' and the income that followed patients from the purchaser to the provider.

---

**Question 4.3**

It has been said that 5 years ago, general practitioners sent Christmas cards to consultants: now consultants send Christmas cards to general practitioners!

Can you explain why this statement helps to illuminate one of the major changes in culture since the NHS reforms became operational?

---

The Government's view of the success of the scheme has led to the further development of it. In April 1996 (the sixth year of the reforms):

- Practices with a population of 5000 may choose to purchase all outpatient attendance and 900 elective medical or surgical procedures from their chosen provider at a known cost
- Practices with a population of 3000 may purchase community services, e.g. health visiting, and direct access services, e.g. pathology
- 49 practices will take the 'total fund'. This follows four pilot projects in which the GP fundholder purchased accident and emergency services, all elective procedures, outpatient attendances and regional speciality activity for their patients

Government targets anticipate that 90% of eligible practices will be fundholding by 1995–96, and that 75% of the population will be served by fundholders by 1996–97. As these general practitioner developments increase, the purchasing role and budget of the Joint Purchasing Health Authorities (DHA/FHSA) will decrease. However, their role in monitoring the GP fundholders and ensuring consistency and achievement of strategic health targets is likely to be enhanced.

## Non-fundholding general practitioners

Some GPs, whether for reasons of small practice size or personal belief, choose not to become fundholders. These GPs are moving to organisations of non-fundholding consortia, ensuring that their views and aspirations for patient care are delivered to the Joint Purchasing Health Authorities (DHA/FHSAs) in a constructive and forceful manner. The outcome of this development is the likelihood of Joint Purchasing Health Authorities receiving purchasing guidance from GPs, which will influence the way the Joint Purchasing Health Authorities place contracts for health care.

---

**Question 4.4**

Will disappointed patients on long waiting lists understand that waiting lists can arise because of purchasers' decisions and funding deficiencies, rather than failure of providers to deliver services?

---

## Providers

Providers consist of any organisations with whom purchasers contract for services and, were given a clear remit in the original reforms to provide high-quality cost-effective care. Common examples include acute hospital trusts, community trusts and private hospitals. This has now developed to include general practitioners themselves, e.g. for minor procedures. The 'NHS trusts' caused most of the initial publicity in the reforms, with hospitals allegedly 'opting out' of the NHS and creating the potential for widespread privatisation. This has not materialised and all remaining directly managed units (DMUs) will by 1996 be self-governing with approved Trust status.

The Trust is governed by the Trust Board, consisting of a chairperson appointed by the Secretary of State, five part-time non-executive directors, usually from business and commerce, and five executive directors, including the chief executive.

---

**Question 4.5**

If non executive directors are drawn from industry and commerce

- What special knowledge and skills could they bring to their role?
- What would be the advantages and disadvantages of having non-executives with former NHS experience?

---

The organisation's contract with purchasers, both Joint Purchasing Health Authorities (DHA/FHSA) and GP fundholders, results in income which funds delivery of services of appropriate quality at a mutually acceptable price. It is without doubt that as general practitioners and purchasers have moved contracts to providers delivering higher-quality or more cost-effective care, a number of providers have lost significant levels of business. The inevitable outcome of this has been several trusts reducing in size or closing entirely and in a number of cases, this has led to mergers of trusts and rationalisation of services.

Probably the most significant factors relating to the re-shaping of the provision of services are:

- The speed with which change has taken place
- The scale of the rationalisation which has taken place as a result of purchaser decisions

---

**Box 4.1**  Regional Offices of the Management Executive

From April 1996, Regional Health Authorities will be replaced by regional offices of the Management Executive – 'ROME'
    The role of the regional offices will be to ensure the Government policies are implemented uniformly and to:

- Agree corporate contracts (an agreement of each DHA priorities and amount of activities to be purchased)
- Monitor purchaser performance
- Maintain an overview of public health status at macro level
- Ensure implementation of national policy e.g. *The Health of the Nation*
- Develop regional targets and transmit these to purchasers
- Monitor trust performances
- Approve strategic and operational plans of purchasers and providers
- Receive business cases for capital schemes from trusts

- The increased utilisation of resources: 'doing more with the same'
- The perceived improvement in measurable quality, e.g. Patient's Charter standards
- The continued political distancing by the Government
- The cultural change, e.g. consultant medical staff attitudes

## Contracts

In order to formalise agreements, purchasers and providers form 'contracts'. Although not legally binding, the 'service agreements' are formal documents agreed between the two parties stating the activity and quality of service to be provided in return for an agreed level of income.

---

**Activity 4.1**

The purchaser is the customer of the provider.
  Think of ways in which a provider trust can encourage the purchaser DHA/FHSA to spend more of its budget on the Trust's services.

---

There are three basic forms of contract, with several variations on a theme.

### Block contract

In its present form, a block contract is an agreed level of finance in return for a specific service. The most common example relates to an accident and emergency service, whereby the cost of providing the service dictates the price. The majority of contracts between major purchasers and providers specify that there will be a level of activity (i.e. patients treated) within certain parameters, including agreed quality standards. Should the 'block of activity' which has been funded be exceeded, then the purchaser and provider will need to reach agreement on how the extra patient services provided will be paid for.

---

**Activity 4.2**

Imagine that a trust receives from Purchaser X £700 000 to fund hip replacement surgery for 1 year. After 9 months the budget has been exhausted. Consider whether the Trust should continue to carry out hip replacements for the rest of the year for Purchaser X's patients.

---

## Cost and volume contract

Increasingly more use of the 'shared risk' contract is being encountered. Purchasers and providers agree a level of activity and a price. Should the activity move above or below the agreed tolerance levels, bands of agreed marginal price increases or decreases step in automatically (Box 4.2).

**Box 4.2**   Cost and volume contracts

| | | |
|---|---|---|
| Overactivity | 106–125 cases | Increase income by 20% of full average cost per case |
| | 101–105 cases | No extra income |
| Agreed level of activity | 100 cases | No extra income |
| | 95–99 cases | No extra income |
| Underactivity | 75–94 cases | Reduce income by 20% of full average cost per case |

## Cost per case

Particularly prevalent in contracts with GP fundholders and for small-volume, high-cost cases, these particular contracts require the purchaser to pay for each individual outpatient attendance, day case or inpatient procedure. Significant financial risk for the provider is encountered in this type of contract and accurate information is required if real costs are to be identified. Providers have difficulty in planning and a high degree of control based on detailed information is required by GP fundholders to ensure that their budget is not overextended (Fig. 4.1).

As significantly more GP practices have moved into fundholding it is certainly not uncommon for major acute trusts to have a portfolio of over 100 contracts of varying types upon which they base their income projections, and hence their workload and staffing levels, for the coming year. Whether or not such financial uncertainty and short-term planning necessarily enhances health-care provision is a matter for debate.

---

**Activity 4.3**

List the disadvantages of an *annual* planning and contracting cycle.
Identify the advantages of a 3-year planning and contracting cycle.

| Purchasers | Providers |
|---|---|
| Assess health needs | Consider purchasing plans |
| Develop purchasing plans | Develop business plan |
| Consult with GP's, providers etc | |
| Develop contract proposals (Quality, activity, price) | Develop contract proposals (Quality, activity, price) |
| Negotiate | Negotiate |
| Form contracts | Form contracts |
| Monitor contracts | Set budgets and deliver contracts for patient services. |
| Evaluate impacts and reassess health needs | Evaluate performance and consider new purchasing plans |

**Fig. 4.1** The cyclical contracting process

# MARKETING AND CONTRACTING

## Marketing

The majority of staff employed in the health service prior to 1991 would have stated quite categorically that marketing was not only an alien terminology but one that should have no place in the NHS. Should a survey be carried out in 1996, 5 years into the reforms, there would be, as with most aspects of the health service, a different view, certainly among the enlightened! To understand this changing attitude and the greater acceptance of the term, it is first necessary to understand both the concept and the changed environment in which it is now being embraced.

## The concept of marketing

The historical development of marketing principles can be applied to the way that health services have been provided to the public prior to the recent reforms:

- *Production orientation.* From the development of the printing press by Gutenberg in the 15th century through to the Model T Ford, the principle of continually producing a product irrespective of user/patient opinion can be applied to certain aspects of the health services, where the professional's opinion is the only one that counts.

- *Product orientation.* The principle of 'build a better product and the world will beat a path to your door' can be seen in a variety of National Health Service developments. Examples include the 'perceived better product' being supplied by some of the London teaching hospitals prior to the reforms.

- *Sales orientation.* The adage 'we will sell what we want to make' is the principle applied in this model. Once again it is possible to apply this to some hospitals early in the reforms. There was a belief that the services available would be accepted anyway, and customers, particularly GPs, would have to accept what was offered, having little say in cost or quality of outcome.

- *Marketing orientation.* The principle is that it is not what you want to provide but what your customer wants you to provide that is of paramount importance. As GPs and other purchasers become more discriminating, so providers must adapt their services to meet their needs.

Much of the argument related to which style is likely to be most successful revolves around the question of 'how educated is the customer?' Increasingly, the customers, be they patients, GPs, major purchasers or pressure groups, are more educated and informed with regard to the health service, their rights, their wants, needs and desires, and therefore in the new reformed NHS market 'the customer is king!'

---

**Question 4.6**

Why are the public more informed about their rights as NHS users?
What steps could be taken to raise awareness even more?

---

The division between purchasers and providers has resulted in the 'internal market'. Applying the principle of 'providing the customer with what they want' has been one of the most significant factors in determining the success or failure of providers in the NHS. This has been most dramatically illustrated in the competition for GP fundholder business. Market research into the wants, needs and desires of GPs, changing a hospital's service to meet those purchasing intentions and then delivering the service has produced the successful market leaders.

Early into the reforms, the Wolverhampton Hospitals decided upon a strong marketing strategy. This was developed partly in response to the threat of losing up to £20m income should GPs choose not to continue to send their patients across the boundary into Wolverhampton from neighbouring areas.

Significant management effort was placed into liaising with GPs, their practice managers, nurses and fund managers as well as, most importantly, the patients. This research provided the following and consistent list of requirements:

- Access in terms of short waiting times and locally provided services where possible
- Quality of care
- Clinical excellence
- Enhanced communications between provider units and GPs
- A lasting partnership
- Competitive price and value for money

The strategy, although elaborate in practice, was of simple concept, i.e. investigate what the GPs want and then ensure that it is delivered.

**Box 4.3** Case study – access to outpatient services

Detailed discussions with a geographically distant GP indicated entire satisfaction with the hospital inpatient service and clinical expertise. The major problem in developing the business in Wolverhampton Hospitals revolved around the travelling distance for outpatient consultations. There was clearly a difficulty for patients to travel some 20 miles in order to be met by an unknown member of staff and to receive a relatively short consultation. Other more local hospitals could provide a similar service without the patient having to make the inconvenient journey.

It was agreed that the most sensible solution for Wolverhampton clinicians was to provide the outpatient clinic locally. This followed detailed clinical discussion and careful management to ensure a successful enterprise that did not reduce the services in the hospital base when medical staff were spending time carrying out clinics in GP surgeries.

The success in 'providing the customer with what they want' was clearly illustrated. The market share for the hospital, and resulting income, increased significantly. The customers, both GPs and patients, received a much improved service. This strategy has now been further developed, with some 50 clinics being 'out-posted' into appropriate localities.

## CONCLUSION

Moving towards the internal market has brought significant changes to the National Health Service. The most radical of these changes is the purchaser–provider split and the granting of the fundholding status to GPs. Initially this change was viewed with both scepticism and caution, but a few years down the road it has been seen to cause a fundamental shift of power away from the providers of the service. The GP is now the key player in the health-care arena, with the freedom to contract health care on behalf of his patients with the provider units that best demonstrate value for money. Initially the contracting process between the purchaser and the provider was very experimental but it has quickly matured and with that has come an increased realisation on the side of the GPs as to the power they hold over the providers in their pursuit of the best possible deal for their patients. This power will increase even more as contracting for health care gathers further momentum and as GPs join together to form consortia and cartels in an attempt to flex their purchasing muscles still further. The managed market of health care has brought self-governing status to many acute hospitals and community units and by 1996 it is envisaged that 95% of all acute NHS hospitals will hold Trust status. Self-governing status has brought relative autonomy to hospitals and community units, but coupled to this autonomy is the ever-increasing threat to survival. Before 1990 it was hard to visualise the health service as a market and even more difficult to imagine that hospitals might close through lack of business. However this is now the reality and even should there be a change of Government, the purchaser–provider split seems here to stay.

## REFERENCES

Department of Health 1989 Working for patients. HMSO, London
The National Health Service and Community Care Act 1990. HMSO, London

## FURTHER READING

Boyle S, Harrison A 1995 Wheel and deal. Health Service Journal 105: 24–26
Ham C, Haywood S 1993 The NHS – a guide for members and directors of health
  authorities and trusts, 2nd edn. National Association of Health Authorities and
  Trusts (NAHAT), Birmingham
Holliday I 1992 The NHS transformed. Baseline Books, Manchester
Hunter D 1995 The purchaser/provider split – is it fatally flawed? Health Director
  18: 17
Lilley R 1993 Trust management and strategy. 101 questions for the board. Radcliffe
  Medical Press, Oxford
Oakley P, Greaves E 1995 A catalyst for change. Health Service Journal 105: 30–31
Ranade W 1994 The future for the NHS – health care in the 1990s. Longman, Harlow

# Decision-making and problem-solving

*Jennifer Clark*

The modern organisation involves numerous decisions made daily by managers; in fact the typical image of management is one of rapid decision-making, the quality of which determines the success or failure of the organisation. The good manager is identified as one who makes clear, timely and correct decisions and the right to make decisions within an organisation is linked closely to status and power. This status is usually much sought after by those with upward career aspirations. The media is keen to reinforce this image and is often guilty of romanticising decision-making by portraying the manager as someone who deals competently and calmly with decisions, the correctness of which brings ultimate glory.

In reality, however, decision-making is less glamorous, but nevertheless remains a very crucial part of the manager's role. Research studies into the characteristics of effective leadership identified the ability to solve complex problems and make decisions as a common trait demonstrated by the majority of effective leaders (see Table 1.3). It is therefore important that this management text addresses the issue of making decisions and solving problems and offers the reader some guidelines for developing this essential skill. Before embarking on this process, however, it is important to differentiate between decision-making and problem-solving and to examine their inter-relationship.

*Organisational decision-making* is the process of choosing actions that are directed towards the resolution of organisational problems. (Mitchell 1982)

*Decision-making* is the process of choosing a course of action for dealing with a problem or opportunity. (Schermerhorn et al 1991)

We see *decision-making* as focusing around the central problem of choice between courses of action. *Problem-solving* is a broader process which includes the recognition that problems exist, the interpretation and diagnosis of that problem and the later implementation of whatever solution is thought to be appropriate. (Cooke & Slack 1991)

Confusion currently exists between the two terms. This confusion has arisen from the tendency of managers to interchange them, thus suggesting that they mean the same thing. However, the above definitions suggest to us that the two are inter-related rather than synonymous, with decision-making being used within the problem-solving process. Problem-solving involves several stages of which the selection of the most appropriate solution from a range of solutions is one. It is within this process of choice that decision-making features.

## THE CONTEXT OF PROBLEM-SOLVING/ DECISION-MAKING

Managers do not solve problems and make decisions in isolation, they are influenced by the environment in which they work and the role that they fulfil within that environment. Schermerhorn et al (1991) identify three types of decision environments encountered by managers:

- Certain environments
- Risk environments
- Uncertain environments

**Certain environments.** This is the most comfortable of the three environments in which to make a decision, but unfortunately it is the environment least often encountered. In certain environments managers are in receipt of sufficient information to allow them to select the best solution, by being able to predict exactly the results of each alternative prior to implementation.

**Risk environments.** This is the environment most often encountered by managers when making decisions and it describes the environment in which the manager lacks complete certainty as to the outcome of different courses of action, but is aware of the probabilities that could occur. These probabilities are sometimes estimated using mathematical techniques, (see mathematical modelling, p 118), but it is more likely that the manager uses her/his own experience or intuition to estimate the likely risk associated with her/his choice of action.

**Uncertain environments.** This is the least comfortable environment in which to make a decision. Here the manager is almost forced to make a decision blind. S/he is unable to forecast the possible outcomes of alternative courses of action and therefore has to rely heavily on creative intuition and the educated guess to reach a decision.

## The managerial role

Earlier in the chapter decision-making and problem-solving was emphasised as a crucial role performed by the manager and in fact seen by some as the 'essence of management'. Mintzberg (1973), however, in his summary of the evidence into how managers spent their time, de-emphasised the decision-making role and suggested that managers performed three equally important roles: interpersonal, informational and decisional.

An understanding of these roles is important if we are to place managerial decision-making and problem-solving into its correct context.

### Interpersonal roles

These roles are involved with the formal authority given to managers and the interpersonal relationships that arise from this authority. There are three types of interpersonal role:

- *Figurehead*. Representing the organisation at functions and ceremonies and carrying out duties associated with her/his status
- *Leader*. Acting as role model for others to follow – the provider of direction and guidance – inspiring others to achieve
- *Liaison*. Acting as the link between the organisation and groups and individuals outside of the organisation – developing an effective network

### Information roles

The manager, by nature of her/his formal position of authority is required to collect and disseminate information. There are three types of informational role performed by the manager:

- *Monitoring.* Seeking information relevant to the organisation, so that opportunities and ideas may be identified and threats detected
- *Disseminating.* Passing on information to others to ensure a knowledgeable workforce
- *Spokesperson.* Making a representation to external bodies on behalf of the organisation – the transmission of information outwards into the environment

### Decisional roles

The manager is required to make decisions and solve problems; these roles directly relate to the informational roles as managers acquire information as a result of decision-making. There are four types of decisional role:

- *Entrepreneur.* The manager creates an innovative environment and initiates change; the manager recognises problems and identifies opportunities and decides how these will be effectively handled
- *Disturbance handler.* The manager manages and resolves both potential and actual conflict situations
- *Resource allocator.* The manager decides how the scarce resources of the organisation may be fairly allocated
- *Negotiator.* The manager negotiates with other bodies outside the organisation and makes decisions accordingly; these negotiations may be with the unions over industrial relations issues or with potential customers or suppliers

Within their decisional roles managers have to make decisions about how to deal with problems as they become apparent. Torrington et al (1989) suggest that managers have the following choices open to them:

- *To deal with the problem.* Usually managers will choose to deal with the problem themselves after collecting relevant information.
- *To pass it on.* The manager may decide that s/he is not the appropriate person to deal with the problem and will pass it on either to her/

his superior or to a subordinate, depending on the nature of the problem.

- *To take advice.* The manager may defer dealing with the problem until s/he has taken advice from a reliable source.

- *To set up a working party.* Complex problems may necessitate the corporate consideration of a group of people before a solution can be found. Managers may therefore be tempted to set up a working party; however it is important to stress that protracted discussions over problems in today's climate could result in the organisation becoming too unresponsive to the market. Small task force groups with a short time scale for response have been found to be the most efficient form of group problem-solving in effective organisations (Peters & Waterman 1982).

- *To employ an expert consultant.* Some problems may demand the input of an expert with specific knowledge or experience to assist in the generation of solutions. As consultant advice is usually costly to the organisation their role should be clearly defined from the outset of their appointment.

- *To ignore the problem.* It is generally an unwise strategy to ignore problems when they become apparent. Problems have the tendency to become crises if left undealt with. However, it may be a wise policy for the manager to prioritise problems into those that require immediate attention (i.e. the red-light group) those that require attention as soon as possible (i.e. the amber-light group) and those that can be safely left (i.e. the green-light group). Some problems do have the habit of solving themselves if left undealt-with, but the decision to leave a problem requires careful informed consideration.

The above narrative demonstrates to us that in practice managers make either individual decisions, consultative decisions or group decisions. These decisions can also be either routine or creative decisions.

**Routine decisions** arise in response to common problems occurring within the workplace. These routine problems have been encountered before by managers and through experience they will make a pre-agreed decision. Many such decisions are already established within an organisation by agreed policies and procedures. An example of a routine decision could be to seek three quotes from potential suppliers for a piece of capital equipment in line with the organisation's financial procedures.

**Creative decisions** arise from the need to solve non-routine problems. These problems have not been encountered before and therefore need a degree of imagination and ingenuity in their solution. It is these types of decisions that managers spend much time on, for they require careful consideration and information gathering. Past experience of similar problems may aid the decision-making process, but there is the obvious need of ensuring that the decision is right in the current climate.

To further our understanding of the types of decisions faced by managers, Cooke & Slack (1991) suggest that management decisions can be differentiated by the use of three dimensions, as follows:

**Strategic or operational.** These decisions centre on the degree of involvement of the organisation. Strategic decisions involve the future of the whole organisation and as they encompass a large part of the organisation they are of the utmost importance, they cannot be classified as routine and are usually decided by top management. Operational decisions involve sections of the organisation, they are more mundane in nature, are involved with the daily functioning of the organisation and can sometimes be classified as routine.

**Structured and unstructured.** This dimension classifies decisions by the degree of definition associated to them. A structured decision is clearly defined and easily discernible, while unstructured decisions lack clarity, are poorly understood and are difficult to make.

**Dependent and independent.** Decisions within this dimension are categorised by their degree of dependence on other decisions. The dependence of a decision may be influenced by decisions previously made by the organisation or alternatively by the consideration of future decisions. The dependence of a decision may also be influenced by other decisions occurring within other departments of the organisation. For example, the decision to buy a new computer network for the administration department may depend upon: the past decisions regarding computer hardware and software utilised by the department and the existing expertise of the administrative staff;

the decision regarding the future information technology needs of the department: and the information technology developments occurring within the rest of the organisation, with which the new system must be compatible.

---

**Activity 5.1**

Recall three recent decisions that you have made either within your work or home context. Consider each of these decisions in the light of the three dimensions described above by asking the following questions:

- Was the decision strategic or operational?
- How structured was the decision?
- How dependent was the decision?

---

## THE PROCESS OF DECISION-MAKING AND PROBLEM-SOLVING

Effective decision-making is not based on 'off the top of the head' thinking, it involves methodical thinking that is systematically organised. Theory related to effective decision-making and problem-solving identifies a problem-solving process which is cyclical in nature and comprises of seven stages. This is presented diagrammatically in Figure 5.1.

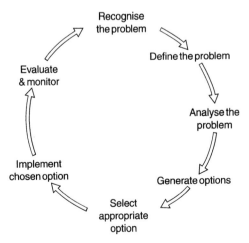

**Fig 5.1**  The problem-solving process (adapted from Stoner 1982)

## Stage 1: Recognition of the problem

This is the first stage in the cyclical process of problem-solving and it involves identifying deficits within the organisation. These deficits exist between what is actually occurring within a given situation (i.e. the actual position or status quo), and what the organisation would like or has planned to be happening (the desired position).

Problem recognition involves two basic aspects. Firstly, the manager must observe and monitor what is going on within the organisation and must be alert to identify deficiencies. The manager will find the goals and objectives of the organisation invaluable in this task. The goals and objectives of the organisation explain its purpose and activity and will act as an effective guide in the determination of discrepancies between what is planned to happen and what is actually happening. Secondly, the manager, after recognising the discrepancy, must evaluate its significance; to do this the manager will need to investigate and to reflect on the situation. This phase within the decision-making process is sometimes referred to as the gestation or incubation period.

## Stage 2: Problem definition

After the problem has been recognised and assessed for its significance it is important to clearly define the problem. Definition of the problem enables the manager to view the problem more clearly and it ensures that in the case of group decisions all members of the group view the problem from the same perspective. In defining the problem it is helpful to first articulate the current situation (actual), then to articulate the situation you would wish to see (desired). The problem can then be defined as the difference between the two positions. Figure 5.2 describes the process.

The definition of the problem should be clear, specific and unambiguous.

---

**Activity 5.2**

Identify a problem from your own work situation and using the process described in Figure 5.2:

- Describe the actual situation
- Describe the desired situation
- Formulate a clear definition of the problem

---

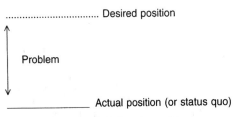

**Fig 5.2** Defining the problem

## Stage 3: Problem analysis

After the problem has been clearly defined it is important to conduct an analysis. Through analysis we develop a clearer understanding of the problem, and this is particularly important when we are dealing with unstructured problems. This stage is often referred to as the information gathering stage, where the manager must assemble information about both the cause of the problem and the possible ways to solve it. Incorporated into this could be the identification of the most suitable people to participate in solving the problem and the type of leadership they will require. The end product of this stage would be an agreed statement of the problem in operational format. This statement should include agreed objectives or goals, the achievement of which would provide the necessary solution.

## Stage 4: Option generation

The next stage of the process is to formulate options that have the potential to solve the problem. The more complex or unstructured the problem the more likelihood there is of generating more options. The generation of plausible options requires both experience and creativity. Brainstorming is a process that is known to foster creative thinking and can be used quite effectively to generate options. This is dealt with more fully later on in this chapter. It is important not to evaluate the options as they are generated as this can seriously hinder creative decision-making, but to allow all suggestions to enter the decision arena before any attempt is made to evaluate and prioritise.

---

**Activity 5.3**

Using the problem identified in Activity 5.2, devise targets or goals that would corporately provide a solution to the problem.

---

## Stage 5: Option evaluation and selection

This is the stage of choice, the selection of the most appropriate option. Option appraisal involves determining which option best fulfils the goals and objectives you have identified in Stage 3. Each option should be considered for its positive features and for its negative features and it is possible to use both qualitative and quantitative data in this process. Options may be costed if the nature of the problem requires this and a scoring system may be devised to facilitate a more objective selection process. At the end of this stage it should be possible to select the option that stands ahead of the field in its potential to solve the problem.

## Stage 6: Implementation of the chosen option

This stage involves making the chosen option work. It is undoubtedly the most difficult, but the most important part of the problem-solving process. There is a tendency to believe that the problem is solved with the selection of an appropriate course of action, but no problem is solved until that action is successfully implemented. Managers should ensure that appropriate resources are in place and that the persons involved are aware of the necessary action they must take to ensure its implementation.

## Stage 7: Evaluation and monitoring

Evaluation of the implementation is essential, and it necessitates monitoring the effect of the chosen option in solving or reducing the problem. If the problem is solved the process ceases at this point but if the chosen option fails to solve the problem or only partially solves the problem then the process returns to Stage 1 and starts again.

## CREATIVITY IN DECISION-MAKING AND PROBLEM-SOLVING

Creativity is about being imaginative in decision-making. It involves the generation of new and exciting ideas that challenge our established belief patterns and liberates us to develop opportunities.

Creativity is an essential component of effective problem-solving; however many of us do not view ourselves as creative individuals. Our stereotyped view of the creative person is one who paints beautiful pictures, composes musical masterpieces or achieves a scientific breakthrough. Creativity, however, is innate in each one of us; it is not limited to the privileged few, although the ability to be creative depends on each one of us being aware of our creative potential and the tactics we can employ to foster its development. Mackinnon (1978) identified five stages in the creative process:

- Preparation
- Effort
- Incubation
- Illumination
- Verification

**Preparation.** During this phase an attempt is made to frame the problem broadly to allow the consideration of as many alternatives as possible. It is during this stage also that the problem needs to be fully understood and all the associated factors recognised.

**Effort.** During this phase effort is made to solve the problem. This may be successful; if not, frustration and stress normally occur. This frustration may lead to a period of withdrawal or incubation.

**Incubation.** During this phase we leave the problem alone. We may sleep on it or seek diversionary activities. This period of rest or incubation allows the brain to think in a less stereotyped way, to engage in more diverse thinking and to formulate more unusual alternatives.

**Illumination.** This is the stage of enlightenment or insight when we break through to a new understanding of the problem. Some may refer to this as the 'Aha!' experience or all the pieces of the jigsaw coming together at once.

**Verification.** This is the stage of implementation when we make our creative idea happen. This may require a logical analysis to confirm the practicality of the idea and to ensure a good decision has been made.

From previous discussion in this chapter it is clear that managers face a variety of problems in the course of their work. Some problems are easily solved, but others are more complex and are more difficult to come up with a solution. Few of the problems encountered by managers fall into the first category of easy to solve; most are the difficult variety. All problem-solving requires a degree of creativity, but the greater the complexity of the problem the greater need there will be for creative thinking.

The greatest block to creative thinking lies not with the problem, however, but with ourselves and centres on the phenomenon known as the *mind set*. Rickards offers the following definitions of mind set.

> Mind sets are personal perspectives based on past experience.
> (Rickards 1990)

> Mind set is the condition of being over sensitised to some parts of the information available at the expense of other parts; it is an inevitable human condition. (Rickards 1990)

Within problem-solving the mind set can be both helpful and unhelpful. It is obvious that our past experience is essential to us if we are to identify problems in their early stages by recognising the warning signs of impending danger, but the mind set can also be a hindrance by acting as a straightjacket and making us too rigid. We become blinkered in our perception of a problem by too readily assuming similarities with the past. Rickards (1990) describes this situation as one of 'stuckness' and says that 'creativity can be seen as an escape from a dominant mind set'. If a dominant mind set is blocking the problem-solving process it is important to trick the brain out of mental stickiness into more creative thinking.

Diversionary tactics can be utilised to do this and these could include exercise, meditation, relaxation techniques and other non-intellectual activities. These activities can interrupt the vicious circle of events that reinforce the dominant mind set. When problems are encountered our first line of response is to examine strategies based on past experience as a means of solving the problem; when these do not work we tend to try harder and redouble our efforts, but this only reinforces the mind set, blocking still further our ability to come up with a creative solution. At this point we need to be aware of our 'stuckness' and challenge the assumptions that bind us to the past. As a leader it is important to ensure that the climate within the organisation is one that fosters creativity among the workforce. Rickards makes this statement regarding creative organisational environments.

> A poor climate for creativity would be one which leads people to avoid risks, be over critical of new ideas and resist attempts to introduce change. A creative environment would be one in which

people trust each other so that they can take psychological risks of being open and revealing their deeper fears and needs. (Rickards 1990)

---

**Question 5.1**

How creative is the climate of your own organisation?

---

**Question 5.2**

What are the main stumbling blocks to creative thinking in your own organisation?

---

## THE TOOLS OF DECISION-MAKING AND PROBLEM-SOLVING

Creativity is about escaping from a mind set which is blocking the way to finding an innovative solution to a problem. An effective tool for assisting in the process is the technique of lateral thinking.

### Lateral thinking

This technique is based largely on the work of Edward De Bono, who regards thinking as a skill which he defines as: 'the deliberate exploration of experience for a purpose' (De Bono 1984, p. 33). He also provides us with a conceptual framework for creative thinking, which he defines as lateral thinking. Through the analogy of escaping from a hole by digging laterally rather than deeper, De Bono advocates that to escape from our mental blockages we need to restructure our thinking process and to think laterally rather than vertically. He suggests several ways of doing this, the intermediate impossible being one and random juxtaposition being another.

#### The intermediate impossible

In this technique De Bono suggests that we break out from the assumptions of our mind set by the use of an outrageous or improbable idea which logistically and rationally we would reject. By the consideration of this idea and by suggesting modifications which would bring it nearer to reality we release ourselves from our mental blockages.

### Random juxtaposition

In this technique De Bono advocates that we select a new concept at random and apply it to the current situation. An example of this might be to select a word at random from a book or dictionary and let your mind explore ways of triggering new ideas for the current problem. A worked example of this is presented in Box 5.1.

---

**Activity 5.4**

Using the worked example in Box 5.1, select a problem that you are finding hard to solve and using random words selected from a book or dictionary generate some new ideas for solving the problem.

---

## Brainstorming

Brainstorming is a technique for generating new ideas or solutions to problems. As it is fairly frequently practised it will already be familiar to many readers. The technique generally involves a small group of people with a common purpose of solving an organisational problem. To do this they generate a wide range of ideas and throw them into

---

**Box 5.1**  An example of random juxtaposition

*Problem*
Effective and timely communication across the surgical directorate of a NHS trust.

*Words selected at random*

• Nocturnal
• Nod
• Node

*Associated ideas*

• **Nocturnal.** Active at night – night staff have particular communication needs.
• **Nod.** Brief gesture. All communication must be brief and concise.
• **Node.** Point on the branch of a tree from which leaves spring. Key persons should be identified who would be responsible for disseminating information to the workforce.

the arena for consideration. The essential feature of brainstorming, and that which separates it from other idea-generating techniques, is deferment of judgement. The evaluation of the ideas must be kept separate from the generation of ideas to ensure maximum contribution from the group. This postponement of judgement requires careful facilitation by the leader as there is a natural tendency to pass judgement on ideas as they are generated and this inhibits creative thinking. Brainstorming is a relatively quick and simple way of collecting new ideas about a problem, but the deceptive simplicity of the technique should not mask the need for careful planning. Attention should be paid to the selection of the team, their suitability and motivation to participate, the selection of the facilitator and the provision of an appropriate location.

## Mind maps

Mind maps provide a framework for thinking; they give it structure and therefore lessen the effect of personal beliefs and assumptions. Three common examples are:

- The fishbone technique
- Relevance trees or hierarchy of objectives
- Concept maps

### The fishbone technique

The fishbone technique involves constructing a diagram of the problem or idea with the central theme in the middle and the subthemes radiating from it. The finished product is a 'picture' of the problem or idea, portraying graphically the main issues involved. Figure 5.3 provides a worked example.

### Relevance trees or hierarchy of objectives

A relevance tree represents a problem broken down into hierarchical components. A central dominant theme is broken down into component parts, from each of which spring further subcomponents. This technique facilitates the analysis of problems down to the lowest denominator. Figure 5.4 represents a simple example of this technique.

### Concept maps

A concept map assists us to store information in a structured format. The way in which information is stored is unique to each individual.

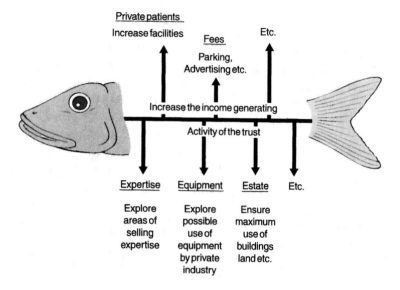

**Fig 5.3**   Fishbone diagram

Over time we formulate our own mental patterns and a concept map represents a visual portrayal of new knowledge using our own specific mental pattern. This technique promotes swift assimilation and recall of knowledge. A worked example of the technique is presented in Figure 5.5.

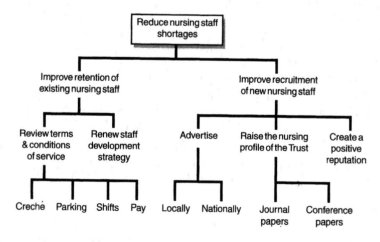

**Fig 5.4**   Relevance tree

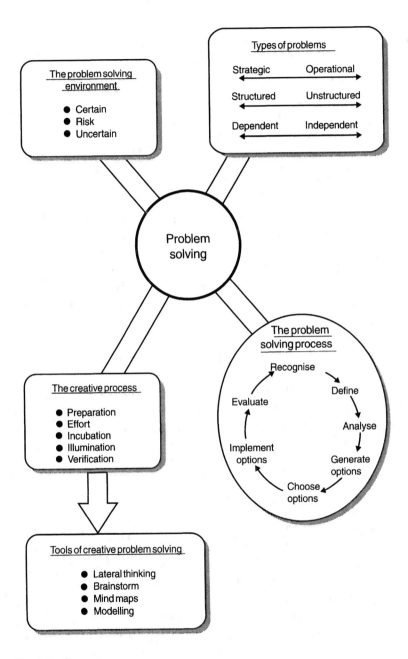

**Fig 5.5** Concept map

**Activity 5.5**

Select a new piece of knowledge that you have recently acquired. Using Figure 5.5 as a guide construct a concept map of that new knowledge.

## Modelling

A model is a visual representation of reality and when used within the process of problem-solving it is a visual statement of the relevant factors involved in the problem. This pictorial portrayal of the problem aids understanding and allows managers to make more informed decisions. As mentioned previously in this chapter, problems are often very complex in nature; associated with them are factors which you can control, but there are also factors that cannot be controlled. Within the modelling process these controllable and uncontrollable factors are called *variables*.

By constructing a representative model of a problem, managers can experiment with different decision options to judge their effect before making the final decision.

Modelling encompasses a wide range of techniques. An example of a very simple modelling technique involves the use of *verbal models*. Managers use verbal models frequently in the process of communicating with their staff. The coordination and reduction of information relating to events in the work place via meetings, team briefings, etc is an example of using a verbal model. At these sessions all subsidiary and non-essential information is removed and the staff are left with a bare profile of the essential facts.

The use of *analogies* is another example of modelling. 'An analogy is the process of arguing similarity in a known respect to similarity in other respects' (*Concise Oxford Dictionary*). The teacher who explains to student nurses that arteriosclerosis can be likened to the furring of water pipes over time is using an analogue model to explain a physiological process. Students can visualise or 'model' the concept in their minds by relating the familiar to the unknown. Graphs and histograms are another way of managers relaying complex information succinctly and clearly. It is easier to explain the relationship between two variables by a graph to an audience than by elaborate description.

As previously stated a model is a representation of reality. It attempts to explain in simple terms how a segment of reality works and operates. A good example of this is the *cause-and-effect model*. The cause-and-

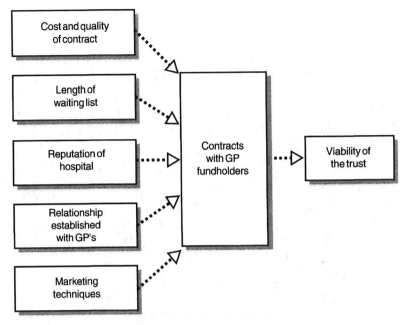

**Fig 5.6** Cause and effect model

effect model aids decision-making by indicating the relationship between different elements of a decision as a simple flow diagram. This is explained in Figure 5.6.

A more complex example of modelling within decision-making is mathematical modelling. In order to develop a mathematical model all the variables within the situation must be able to be measured and expressed in a quantitative form. Harrison (1995) identifies six steps in the construction of a mathematical model.

1. Define the problem and quantify the expected results of the solution (the *dependent variable*)
2. Identify the causes of the problem, especially those that will influence the result; these causes should also be expressed in quantitative form (the *independent variables*)
3. Determine the casual connections between the problem and the results; quantify these connections (this could be done by weighting probability)
4. Create a numerical equation that reliably expresses the relationship between the causes (independent variables) and the result (dependent variables)

5. Test the reliability of the model by substituting actual data from the real world for the independent variables and by observing the effects on the dependent variable; are there differences between what the model predicts and those being experienced in reality?
6. Revise the model by altering the independent variables until the desired dependent variable is obtained

*Computer simulation* is another type of modelling, which has recently become an effective contribution to decision-making. By creating a situation of virtual reality on the computer, managers can use simulation to test out the effects of the different options open to them. Simulation offers the following advantages to decision makers:

• It allows for experimentation with different solutions and allows managers to evaluate and predict the outcome of decisions without risk
• It provides the means whereby the probability of success of an option can be evaluated with minimal time and effort
• It increases the managers understanding of operational systems and thus creates an awareness of possible improvement or development

## CONCLUSION

Problem-solving and decision-making are a crucial part of the manager's role. The process of problem-solving includes the selection of a chosen course of action from a variety of alternatives; it is this element of choice that constitutes decision-making. The environment in which the manager works and the role that s/he fulfils within that environment will influence the way in which s/he makes decisions, as will the nature of the decision to be made – whether it is routine or creative, structured or unstructured. In situations of complexity managers should be aware of the need to be imaginative and to break from the restrictions of their mind set by using creative thinking techniques. The techniques of lateral thinking, brainstorming, mind mapping and modelling are all useful tools to the manager in formulating and testing new ideas.

## REFERENCES

Cooke S, Slack N 1991 Making management decisions. Prentice Hall, London

De Bono E 1984 Teaching thinking. Penguin, Harmondsworth

Harrison E F 1995 The managerial decision making process, 4th edn. Houghton Mifflin, Boston

Mackinnon D W 1978 In search of human effectiveness. Creative Education Foundation, Buffalo, NY

Mintzberg H 1973 The nature of management work. Harper & Row, New York

Mitchell T 1982 People in organisations. An introduction to organisational behaviour. McGraw-Hill, London

Peters T J, Waterman R H 1982 In search of excellence. Harper & Row, London

Rickards T 1990 Creativity and problem-solving at work. Gower, Aldershot

Torrington D, Weightman J, John S K 1995 Effective management, people and organisation. Prentice-Hall, London

Schermerhorn J, Hunt J, Osborn R 1991 Managing organisational behaviour. John Wiley & Sons, Chichester

Stoner J A F 1982 Management, 2nd edn. Prentice Hall, London

# Change in the NHS: strategies and prospects

*Kevin Hogan*

**6**

## ■ CONTENTS

## IDENTIFYING THE PROBLEM

Another chapter with advice on how to manage change needs an explanation in the current climate. Managers in the NHS have had something of a surfeit of change (Working Paper 10) and advice on how to manage it (Caines 1994, McKeown 1995, Spurgeon & Barwell 1991) in recent years. The advent of resource management, the development of the internal economy for health care and the rapid spread of trust status and GP fundholding constitute almost as much change to the system of health delivery in the UK as did the birth of the NHS in 1948. There are many authors who have criticised the basis of the current round of change: the ideological origins of the changes and the logic of these developments, particularly the question of whether or not such changes can deliver an improvement in quality and value for money from the service. Also, the manner in which the changes have been managed has not escaped scrutiny. As an original contribution to the debate this chapter is designed to explore the nature of change, to describe some changes as they are unfolding in the NHS and to make suggestions in the light of the literature on organisational change and innovation. The main focus will be to discuss the nature of change such that attempts to manage the process can be driven by an understanding as rich and complex as the process itself.

Much of what is written about change describes change as an object, a discrete entity, a thing in its own right, usually loosely characterised as a process, that has to be managed by somebody or some group of people. From this point of view the question of what to do about change is relatively straightforward – change is a process we all know about in some common sense way, but which needs to be clearly structured and understood so that it can be managed. This is the problem that this chapter is designed to address.

Change is not a single process or group of processes: in a very important sense, 'it', that is to say change, does not exist at all. It is an ideal, a story made by everyone who is experiencing a discontinuity. Viewed by some as a cause for events, by others as a consequence, it can be the disease, the diagnosis and the cure. Organisations, individuals, managers, academics, doctors, nurses – indeed, in this day and age, everyone on the Clapham omnibus including the driver – has a view as to the importance and endemic nature of change. Like stress, and indeed often linked with stress, change is commonly understood as a form of modern organisational disease.

Change suffers from another problem like stress: in the research literature and in practice it has a bewildering variety of definitions. Each of these definitions is in effect a theory of change. In practical terms a theory is, in the hands of those faced with practical problems, a device that allows the manager to do three things: predict the future on the basis of a theory and knowledge of the present circumstances, control the situation and finally make sense of or understand what it is that is actually happening. All three of these derive from having an effective theoretical understanding of what the organisation is experiencing. This chapter is designed to promote a practical theory of change and change management that will help achieve all three of these goals. It is based on the fundamental premise that employees need to make sense of their working lives, invest heavily in work and apply a sense of justice to the experience.

## WHAT IS 'CHANGE'?

Change as an experience is different for the originator and the recipient of change, for the manager and the managed, for the organisation that originates it from within its own boundaries (endogenous change) and for the company or organisation upon which change is somehow inflicted, as it were (exogenous change). At each level of a business and in differing sets of circumstances the threats and opportunities afforded by change will differ and differ dramatically. In point of fact the first major point about change is that even in circumstances where a single objective event would seem to be 'the change', for example where a group of hospitals amalgamate and take trust status, the fact is that for a whole host of entities within the new organisation, from departments to individual employees, a whole galaxy of change(s) will be experienced. The issue here is that change is not a single event or action and where it is treated as such this may lead to misconceived interventions and missed opportunities. By way of illustration, consider the well known problem of maintaining staff commitment at times of organisational change. Commitment is 'the product of more than just structural arrangements: something is necessary to breathe life into formal organisational relationships and to make actual what structure only makes possible' (Hales 1993, p 188).

## A HOLISTIC APPROACH TO MANAGING CHANGE

Hales recommends that in approaching the problem of developing and maintaining commitment a holistic approach is required. The rich web of interdependencies and patterns of connectivity that characterise organisations, he argues, must militate against a 'piecemeal approach'. This argument concerning commitment must be extended to the management of change. A holistic approach involves the recognition that organisations contain human agents who actively try to make sense of and exploit opportunities presented by change stimuli. The alternative perspective, where attention is focused on objective change events, requires that managers identify any and all aspects of the business affected by change and explicitly organise the response of the organisation at all levels – or ignore them. In practice what this often means is that those aspects of change that are suited to the values, interests, capabilities, skills and experience of managers are focused upon and in some limited sense managed. However, aspects of change that are not congruent with the management culture will not be integrated into the pattern of explicit responses made by the organisation. As an example of this we have the recent evidence that one factor in the very high rate of failure for mergers and acquisitions is the tendency of management planning such changes to focus on technical and financial aspects of the planned integration at the expense of examining the potential conflict in terms of merging two dissimilar social cultures (Cartwright & Cooper 1994). It is apparent from the research literature that failures very frequently arise from an incompatibility between the two organisational cultures in mergers and acquisitions. It is necessary to understand that organisational culture is a major variable to be addressed when managing change. The point here, however, is that whereas managers can understand the technical issues associated with change, or retain consultants who can, it is more frequently the case that other issues raised by change go by the board because they are outside the range of competencies of the staff involved.

A second problem arising from the conceptualisation of change as a discrete event is that, if management make the mistake of attempting to manage all aspects of change in a rational and pre-planned way (although there is much evidence that often change management is neither rational nor pre-planned), then problems arise when the complex of reactions and re-actions that progress like waves outwards from the sites of change leads to new strategies, structures and operating behaviours which in turn have unintended consequences that might well need managing. The unintended consequences of Departments A's new operating strategy will quickly force a change in the behaviour of Department B; this in turn may well need new developments in the functioning of Department A or indeed include effects further afield at Department C. All of this will be compounded by the fact that, as we look from the front-line worker to the first line manager/supervisor and then the departmental manager and above, the time period before the effects of change will be detected and a response will need to be formulated increases significantly. For example, at shop floor level the implications of a new change in working practices may be apparent within hours, and certainly within 3 months, while at departmental level this same recognition may take a year to develop, or indeed longer as the recognition of the problem diffuses up the organisation (Anderson & Ginnerup 1992). The implications of this for managing and coordinating are clear – management cannot predict all the consequences of change, nor can they necessarily be identified in time for orderly coordination of responses. Moreover, change is not limited to the immediate time or obvious consequences of a single objective change event.

In line with the view of change developed above, it is clear that change cannot be managed solely at the point of or just before a specific event – change is managed both by acting on a case-by-case basis and by developing an organisation that is capable of continuous adjustment and hopefully innovation. Some authors have argued for the management of change being achieved by developing an organisational culture which can initiate and sustain change. The concept of the learning organisation is a good example of this approach. Certainly, research aimed at developing an understanding of innovation in organisations makes it clear that not all organisations can produce let alone sustain change (West & Farr 1990). Indeed, it has been suggested that for some organisational structures to expect change is foolish in the extreme.

## CREATING A CLIMATE FOR CHANGE

There is agreement in the literature concerning the types of practice and procedure that can foster effective change. At the strategic level this involves the consistent attempt over time to build up trust between the various constituencies within the organisation. Every attempt at organisational change takes place in the context of the relationships and history established by the prior records of all parties involved in earlier change events. Thus a key component in the effective management of change is the creation of a climate for change which foreshadows mutual respect, significant advance notice of change intentions and the prospect of meaningful negotiations concerning these, concepts frequently enshrined in legislation governing the workplace abroad, e.g. in France and Sweden. At this level it is apparent what kind of task faces NHS management. What might be considered the preconditions for successful planned and centrally directed change are not in place. Moreover some aspects of the changes in hand, which will be discussed below, actually militate against achieving these preconditions. The creation of new operational entities setting aside institutional histories and fracturing pre-existing loyalties and shared understandings allows individuals to reconsider or set aside the framework of obligations that once governed their work (see the discussion of the psychological contract, below). At the same time this lack of an organisational history means that mutual trust and respect has to be made and earned at exactly the moment when management may well need to rely on it to carry the organisation through trying times.

## THE POLITICAL CONTEXT

Continuing at the strategic level of analysis, let us briefly take a look at the political goals underpinning the move for change in the NHS, remembering that a key aspect of change management strategy is to 'sign up' those affected by either a) representing their diagnosis of a need to change and ideas as to the content of change or b) recruiting them to the perception of the problem and its resolution offered by the management. If the staff of the NHS had been asked to prioritise their change efforts in the last years of the 20th century, beset as the service is by demographic and technical changes on a large scale, would they have placed the transfer of workload and responsibility for financial and operational management to the medical staff at the top of their list? I think not and yet this move is a political reality; the government of the day believes that market economics can regulate the operation of the NHS in a way that central government has failed to do despite numerous large-scale reorganisations since 1948. Market disciplines, it is hoped, will provide the framework within which costs can be controlled and quality managed by the invisible hand of competitive forces. At the same time it is also a reality that if a workforce does not subscribe to the values and goals implicit in any new strategy then managing the change process will be that much more difficult. It would be naive in the extreme to set out in the last years of the 20th century to manage a large and relatively highly skilled workforce on the premise that they will do what they are asked to do, in the spirit of that request, simply because they are paid to do so. Indeed, we can be certain that such would not be the case, if only because of what we have learned about the sociology of the professions, particularly medicine – or perhaps from the experience of a similar approach and its consequences when applied to the education service in recent years (Ranson 1994).

It would appear that a related difficulty with the implementation of change in the NHS has been the lack of a clear set of ethical principles underpinning the marketisation of the NHS, a clear professional identity for the instigators or indeed a coherent mission to serve as focus for their work (Haggard 1993). This makes their job of altering work practices, changing attitudes and the balance of power at work all the more difficult.

## THE IMPACT OF MARKET FORCES

One aspect of the move (or return) to market forces as a disciplinary framework for the NHS has been the reintroduction of local pay bargaining. Although currently restricted to the low-paid (low-power) groups of workers, these reforms do not augur well for the stability of the industrial relations scene or the prospect of a smooth path to organisational change. Unions such as those representing nurses in the NHS are tremendous stabilising influences; it is true that, from some perspectives at least, they appear as a significant brake on the rate of change. But with the loss of institutional inertia so too will the degree of consensus governing people's approach to work breakdown and factionalism will come to the fore. The task of managing the factions that emerge and binding together the new organisations will fall to those charged with managing a far more unstable industrial relations scene. Moreover, as the current wave of uncertainty and redundancies dies away and the move to a more flexible workforce, employed on a variety of contracts, comes into play, the negotiating position of the NHS vis a vis staff, in some specialties in particular, will be a difficult one and wage inflation can be expected in some quarters at least. In the short term, multiple constituencies of skilled, particularly specialised and organised staff may well come to represent a source of conflict and not consensus as the NHS changes.

As contracts of employment increase in number and complexity then so too do those contracts binding trusts to consumers of their services. Of necessity these contractual relationships will give rise to two different classes of effect that will need to be looked at. We will see, as is already emerging, that many thousands of purchase and employment contracts create a new form of labour within the organisation. The work involved is not directly related to the delivery of the service that justifies the existence of the institution and it is complex and therefore requires trained and well paid staff. Thus resources will be diverted in a highly visible fashion into 'non-productive' activities. This will in itself cause problems because unless handled very carefully such a change will not meet with widespread understanding and approval. At the local level, i.e. within a department in a trust hospital, this type of work will be increased as the unit of accounting becomes even smaller. Some trusts have, for example, taken the marketplace model and reapplied it to the internal organisation of the organisation. Thus some hospitals are creating an internal market where each operational unit is being put into the business of selling its products, be they goods or services, to other parts of the same and similar organisations. One effect will be a widespread and continuing demand for administrative staff at the same time as rationalisation is taking place in the staffing levels of other operational groups.

## DATA COLLECTION AS A BARRIER FOR CHANGE

A second effect poses difficulties for the smooth management of change – quite simply, the increased and collective burden of counting and accounting for the activities involved in service delivery in immense (new) detail. In the main such tasks will fall on existing staff who do not see themselves as administrators. Notwithstanding the logical status of such activities, forming as they do the very essence of the market-led approach to a disciplined health service, the organisation of and rationale for such activities will need to be handled very carefully. Experience with organisational change driven by computer technology points to just this class of activities as a point of tension. Firstly, unless those enjoined to collect or input the data are very clear about why they are undertaking such activity – i.e. they appreciate both the reason for and the use made of the information they handle – problems can be expected. If highly trained staff faced with multiple demands on their time and a clear sense of professional and ethical responsibility have to prioritise their work, then 'meaningless clerical work' cannot be expected to claim their full attention. Data can be adjudged meaningless because in the view of the professional it is 'wrong', or misleading because it is asking the wrong questions, at the wrong time or place. These views should not arise when a) the data to be collected is discussed with staff in the first place and/or b) they are fully briefed as to the significance of the data. If the significance of the information collected is not clear then experience suggests that avoidable errors in data collection will arise because the data input will be being carried out by someone who does not understand the implications of their actions. In a number of areas no data, or at least not enough data, will be collected in the first place. These effects will not be uniform: it can be expected that functions that impinge on professional standing, such as quality assurance statistics, will not be collected as assiduously as data that have a more direct impact on service provision.

In short, in many areas the new work may well be adjudged to be a further burden on under-resourced staff. It is essential that this is avoided by developing and implementing such changes in an inclusive fashion. The goal must be to develop information acquisition and retrieval systems which are valued by those who enter the data as well as those who process it and to develop such systems with the rules of sound ergonomic (Singleton 1989) and human-centred system designs principles (Eason 1988). What this should mean in practice for example is that wherever possible data acquisition techniques should be employed that minimise the overheads for collection and data entry. Thus hand-held bar code scanners should be adopted in preference to having clinical staff typing data into terminals. When questionnaires are designed they are cheap to produce and distribute and the cost of each one is represented by the work of the respondent in filling it out. Attention should be given to alternatives: sampling systems using interviews or focus groups, accessing the data from other sources and the use of on-line questionnaires.

Whatever the merits of this increase in the accounting for activities in the service, it cannot fail to impinge on many staff in the new market-driven NHS. In almost every field significant amounts of staff time will be required to make the new systems required by the market operate. As budgets become smaller and more tightly focused, as customers such as GP fundholders require that records are kept regarding the fate of 'their' patients, waiting time, costs of diagnosis and treatment, outcomes, evaluations, all these and more will cut across the judgement and autonomy of professionals hitherto relatively unencumbered by such considerations. At least, that is, unencumbered by the need to supply such information as a matter of course and to people outside their professional orbit and host institution. Where the benefit of the extra work of data collection and data handling is not immediately obvious or, worse still, is seen to impinge on the autonomy and authority of those charged with managing the collection of it, problems can be anticipated. Emphasis must be placed upon developing a sense of ownership, focused as far as possible by the sense that information collected is both owned by and at the disposal of those who collect it.

## THE IMPORTANCE OF DATA MANAGEMENT

In order to foster effective change, new data collected must be available at the right time, in an understandable and useful format and in such a form that the overheads associated with retrieval and analysis do not prevent the users from actually exploiting it. It is all too frequently the case that data management is confined to the timings and formats that meet the needs of the various audit requirements. If at all possible, multiple uses need to be identified and built into the information management system so that all potential constituencies affected by or contributing to the data set can fully exploit the resource. For example an outpatient clinic may well use a properly constructed data set as a research resource; in any event the data should be made available to the clinic as a matter of course in a way that suits their needs. Failure to follow this approach invites the view that systems that are 'not invented here' need not be supported or used because the data and the problem belong to someone else. As part of the process of change management the commitment of data users and data providers is essential in order to achieve the high levels of efficiency that such systems ought to reach to justify the investment they represent. This can only be achieved in the final analysis if all potential users exploit the system to the full; this requires commitment and not a control approach.

## MULTISKILLING PROFESSIONAL PRACTITIONERS

Another aspect of change driven in this fashion is the transfer of responsibilities and skills between professions. So-called 'empowerment' or 're-engineering' becomes a method for multiskilling the practitioner. A senior nurse becomes a manager with multiple budgetary and personnel responsibilities. The practice of her/his professional skills becomes less and less the focus of her/his attention. Similarly, a doctor faced with a new organisational structure, budgetary and management tasks may begin to lose sight of research interests. Such developments are all too common and the costs for the individual and the organisation can be serious if the new roles do not allow for job satisfaction and the organisation provides inadequate support, either by virtue of the organisational design or training and resource allocation. To go from concentrating on activities that can be immensely rewarding and in respect of which the individual feels confident of her/his own abilities to activities that appear to offer only the potential for failure and loss of self-confidence does not bode well for effective change.

---

**Activity 6.1**

Consider a change shortly to be implemented within your own work situation. What action had been taken to facilitate its smooth implementation?

---

## INNOVATION

In order to foster effective change in advance of particular events or circumstances an organisation must lay the groundwork for innovation; the ability to initiate and incorporate successful change is a critical factor in terms of success in a changing environment. Innovation can be defined as the adoption of an idea or behaviour that is new to the adapting organisation (Daft 1982). A point made by Damanpour (1990) is that it is change new to the organisation that is of interest: a new system, device, policy, process, program, product or service – not simply 'new ideas'.

Innovatory behaviour can be thought of as the explicit search for productive change; a proactive rather than a reactive approach to change management. Innovatory change is the attempt to modify behaviour, products, processes or procedures in order to enhance the effectiveness of an organisation. Innovatory change is not necessarily a response to a diagnosis highlighting problems but rather a technique, or set of techniques, for identifying or indeed 'manufacturing' opportunities for change. The major focus of interest in innovation in the business/management and educational development psychology literature has taken two forms: 'the development of creative talents within individuals, and the process of innovative product development within manufacturing concerns' (Anderson 1992).

At base this view of innovation is about performance: innovatory behaviour is the ability to add value in whatever context. Recently in the industrial and organisational literature some attempt has been made to integrate these approaches into a framework in which innovation has been studied at the organisational, group and individual level (Hosking & Anderson 1992). At the same time, innovation has been described as a management strategy for coping with and indeed creating change (Peters 1989). It has been argued that environmental change in particular requires organisational innovation; managing such innovation has become a key aspect of strategic thinking (Anderson 1992). The effective businesses will be those which can foster a climate supportive of innovation. In effect an innovatory organisational climate can be thought of as fostering problem-solving behaviour in advance of the diagnosis of specific problems. This proactive stance has been identified by several authors as a source of significant competitive advantage in companies pursuing such a strategy (Senge, 1990).

## ENVIRONMENTAL INFLUENCES

It is almost a commonplace observation that major public and private sector organisations increasingly have to manage in a turbulent and competitive environment. The NHS is a particular example in that not only has the external environment in which the service operates changed dramatically in recent years, but the central thrust of recent reforms have been to put in place mechanisms that ensure that new competitive forces will hold sway for the first time in decades. Such forces will not only act to create change but more importantly will increase the rate of change within the service. The need to manage change arises not solely from the requirement to incorporate the new market disciplines into management strategy, but also from the need to build organisations capable of constant and indeed accelerating change. The implication of competition is not 'now we must compete' but rather 'now we must all be prepared to change to gain a competitive advantage'. The consequence of this kind of behaviour is to create instability (competition), which must lead to further change in response to changing circumstances.

In the context of pressure to sustain and indeed create constant change, contingent issues such as adoption or diffusion rates come to the fore. A model of innovation that views organisations as a user of innovation poses the question: why do some organisations adopt an innovation more frequently or readily than other organisations? The question of how a particular innovation spreads in an organisation or group of organisations, in other words what is the process of diffusion, must also be examined.

## STRUCTURE, CULTURE AND CLIMATE

The relationship between organisational structure, culture, climate and innovation with respect to their impact upon the success of organisations in adopting innovations and diffusing them throughout a business warrants consideration. In his anti-mechanistic or organic model of innovative organisations, Nystrom (1990) has made it clear that he relates successful innovation to both organisational structure and culture. Although different structures can have their (relative) value, the innovative division or company will have a more organic structure and innovative culture, in effect it is the self-actualising organisation.

One could propose a model that sets aside the notion of top-down control, where innovations spread from the top of an organisation and innovation is seen as a standard business process whereby central control is exercised. Control could be seen as the emergent property of the coupling between a commercial entity and its environment. In this respect, innovation requires that we recognise that we cannot know exactly what will happen or how, a problem area in which the unknowable aspect of many decisions is recognised.

Innovation and productive change cannot be 'made' to happen: successful change is the function of a host of properties of a complex system; the aim can be to foster the circumstances, training, organisation structure, culture and strategy that can foster and sustain change.

It must be remembered that the communication processes inside an organisation, including the symbolic representation of the organisation

**Box 6.1**

Culture = the values, norms, beliefs and assumptions held in common within an organisation.
Climate = feelings, attitudes and behavioural tendencies.

to itself (see below), are a significant manifestation of 'control' within that organisation. For example, a humanistic philosophy underpinning recruitment policy will constrain the wide range of potential ways in which management might select staff; it will also become part of the way in which new staff come to be aware of the organisational culture.

Nystrom's model of organisational change (1990) describes innovative direction as the nature of the radical changes a company wishes to make. Innovative potential is the ability of the company in terms of its structural constraints, i.e. material and human resources to carry out that change. Strategic leadership is the effort to decide what an organisation can do and what it wants to do as a company.

For Nystrom, company culture and climate revolves around the dichotomy between the positional company, which essentially wishes to continue doing what it is already doing, a company which has neither innovative direction not potential, and the other form of company, which is the innovative kind, an organisational entity whose structure is capable of both fostering and implementing change.

*Positional companies* tend to show clarity in goal and behaviour but are less willing and able to take risks and explore new possibilities. Their cultures and climates are less challenging, playful and lively. They are also less supportive of, and less rich in new ideas.

*Innovative companies* are open in their views and behaviour but also show more internal differences in opinion and greater debate as to what action to take to achieve innovative goals.

## CREATING THE RIGHT CULTURE

To create an innovative culture what is required is a consistency in structure, culture, climate and strategic leadership, developments that reinforce and make possible radical change. It follows from this that those companies that do not have the appropriate form of climate, structure and culture should not be the targets of radical change.

Instead such change efforts should be a) directed to new units explicitly set up for the purpose or b) channelled to those parts of the company or companies that have an appropriate infrastructure for change.

A further set of issues that need to be considered surrounds the question of a division of innovation into technical, administrative and ancillary change. Technical change appears to be both more successful and more frequent (Damanpour 1990) than administrative change. Two effects seem to be at work here: firstly, by virtue of prestige and investment, plus the simple physical symbolism of technical innovation, it is more desirable, measurable and consequently attractive. Secondly, it seems clear that, despite the evidence to the contrary, within organisations a view is held that technical and administrative change occur independently of one another. However, it seems very likely that the two forms of innovation have a far more complex relationship.

It has been suggested (Brunsson 1985) that organisations have an ideology or cognitive schema that effectively constrains the kind of change of which they are capable. Organisations with strong ideologies have elaborated and consistent schemata; thus they are capable of detecting inconsistencies between the internal system and environmental demands. In the strong ideology organisation this will lead to substantive change. By contrast, unarticulated, weak and ambiguous ideology organisations simply absorb the pressure to change, making symbolic rather than substantive responses to the changing circumstances.

## ORGANISATIONS AS 'INTERPRETATIVE SYSTEMS'

Nicholson (1990) briefly noted a concept of organisations as differing in kind and degree as 'interpretative systems'. In effect he argued that the organisational preference for substantive rather than symbolic change would be influenced to a great extent by the nature of the reflective discourse within organisations. In other words, he has argued that to the extent that an organisation can articulate a sophisticated self-concept in terms of symbolic and decision-making activity, it will be more likely to engage in substantive change and evolve into a less self-centred and more self-aware entity. Self-awareness can be construed as a method of enquiry. The self-aware organisation, capable of handling indeterminacy, is an organisation capable of engaging in enquiry and capable of producing and identifying productive change.

## IS THE NHS A SELF-AWARE ORGANISATION?

Given that the National Health Service will from now on be a site for change in almost every aspect of its operations, one new need arises that will become central to strategic management: the requirement to build and remake a sophisticated model of what is happening. This is not solely in terms of the needs and views of its customers and patients – what will also be required is a dynamic picture of what is happening within the service itself. Greater self-awareness and a sophisticated model or self-image is required and it must be subject to constant and rigorous scrutiny. Operational efficiency as identified in accounting terms will not suffice to sustain and develop such a complex and massive undertaking.

## RESISTANCE TO CHANGE

The research literature, commercial publications and the press all point to a very high degree of systems failure associated with the implementation of new computer based business systems (Eason 1988). A similar high rate of damaging failure is associated with take-over or merger activities in all forms of organisation (Cartwright & Cooper 1994). Other writers have pointed out how change is changing, i.e. how organisations are being required to change not in an incremental or evolutionary manner but in revolutionary or disjunctive fashion; 'the idea of disjunctive change is helpful, drawing attention as it does to the problems associated with social upheavals' (Blackler 1992). All these notions serve as guidelines for an analysis of the situation in the NHS where disjunctive change is the order of the day and social

**Box 6.2**

'A critique is not a matter of saying that things are not right as they are. It is a matter of pointing out on what kinds of assumptions, what kinds of familiar, unchallenged unconsidered modes of thought the practices we accept rest . . . criticism is absolutely indispensable for any transformation.' (Foucault, in Kritzman 1988, p 154) upheaval characterises the experience of many employed in the service. Among the reasons for the failure of the change process, the reaction of employees to change is a frequently cited cause (see Willcocks & Mason 1987). In this section a range of possible responses to change, which might be characterised as resistance to change, are discussed.

## Employee resistance

The contention that resistance is the result of incapacity on the behalf of affected staff to comprehend the truth, logic or validity of a new working practice, technologies or organisational structures, is a naive and counterproductive standpoint. It is counterproductive because it encourages the view that the use of coercion is justified to remove the resistance. If staff are understood to be acting from sheer ignorance and foolishness and lack of insight, then that diagnosis lends weight to a solution based on the direct application of power and the use of coercion to resolve problems. The view that management can change attitudes in the workforce is an example of simplistic thinking; attitudes are by no means as plastic as this view would seem to suppose and managers are all to rarely in a position to control the variables that might give them the ability to manipulate the attitudes of their colleagues. Unfortunately, as has been found, this type of management response is of very limited effectiveness. Many modern organisations are far too complex to be able to be served optimally by any but committed personnel. What is required is a view of staff affected by change that does not describe their responses, be they 'good' or 'bad', in terms of resistance or wrong attitude, but rather seeks to understand why they feel the way they do. It is abundantly clear that the most effective way in which to manage resistance to change is to prevent it occurring in the first place.

If an organisation truly changes, it does it not just by changing the job content or work organisation of some of the staff in the organisation, but throughout the whole organisation. The organisation which once employed most or all of the people has gone. The new organisation may well still occupy some of the space, contracts, staff, customers and practices that characterised the old organisation, but it is not the same. This is the kind of change that confronts the NHS. In these circumstances it is rational that people whose understandings and competencies allow them to make investments in and draw rewards from an organisation might wish to see those assets and values reproduced in the new structure. Resistance can be viewed as an accident or an obstruction, but it is also a logical consequence of thinking human agents seeking to continue to make sense of their working lives. Calling this process resistance is something of a misnomer.

## The reality of practical power

A very good alternative explanation of the processes at work in what some have come to describe as resistance can be found in a paper by Salaman & Butler (1990): they attempted to explain why, in certain contexts, managers won't learn. If there is one assumption that seems to have gained wide support in the literature on change, it is the view that managers will have to learn and continue to learn in order to manage change in the current era (Peters 1992). However, innovation can be viewed as a process whereby change is defined, encouraged and controlled in order to best serve the needs of the dominant power group in an organisation (Nicholson 1990). Organisations are essentially political; highly differentiated as they are into specialisms, functions or departments, every hospital is the site of unremitting competition for limited resources. The ability to control budgets, to manage rewards such as pay, staffing levels, research grants or equipment budgets represents the reality of practical power. Such power over resources is allied to prestige and in the NHS almost always located in a steep and very clearly understood hierarchy.

At the heart of Salaman & Butler's analysis lies the simple proposition that managers won't learn because they already have learned a great deal; they have learned about the realities of organisational power: where it lies, what it is used for and how it is used. This knowledge is 'real' and so too is the structural representation of this knowledge. Salaman & Butler used as one example the power invested in a personnel department when they began training managers to use a new appraisal scheme. Firstly, training managers in new methods of relating to their staff clearly indicates that the personnel department commitment to a method outweighs the freedom of managers to choose, including to choose to continue in the way that they may argue 'works' for them. Secondly, in the example given this feeling was reinforced because not only did managers not want to follow the new guidelines, but their main reason for not doing so was they would no longer be able to manage their own staff in a way understood by both parties. Not only was the innovation an imposition, but it was an imposition with a negative impact on the very area of work that it was nominally designed to address. Taking all of this from the perspective of the manager, resistance appears to be rational and training becomes a rite of submission rather than a transfer of skills. It is interesting how frequently training staff are faced with complaints about the changes that the training is serving.

## Maintenance of the status quo

Staff may well not fall into line with new directives concerning racially aware recruitment practices or new staff appraisal procedures, for example, not because they are racist or obstructive but because these new practices disturb a status quo that works. Until new work practices can be seen not to threaten that status quo it is sensible, from some points of view at least, to resist. And if that resistance is not visible, and it need not be (see below), it can threaten the viability of change processes in ways that preclude effective intervention. The core of this

---

**Box 6.3**  Case study: from Salaman & Butler 1990

A seminar programme designed to address potential racial and gender inequalities in recruitment practices failed – in part, at least, because it did not take account of the logic of the existing practices. In the face of emerging social and legal frameworks for governing employment practices, London Fire Brigade managers had to face the end of a lengthy tradition of recruiting men like themselves: from the same background and geographical area, with similar values and preferably with ties to other members of the brigade. This framework for making and remaking the service had worked, literally, for generations. From the perspective of managers this approach had served the service long and well and had been 'outlawed' by people who did not do the job. If one considers the need for the men to work in a team, depending upon one another in extraordinary circumstances and spending long hours in very close proximity, one can readily see how the previous recruitment strategy must have made sense. Simply telling someone to undermine their own safety and social support system (from their point of view) does not necessarily achieve willing acceptance. The unasked question is: how do you knit together a team, develop mutual understanding and confidence if the old ways are abandoned?

---

problem would appear to be the fact that issues such as recruitment practices are deeply embedded in the social, political and hence economic culture of the organisation. It is unfortunate that change by fiat, in the case study in Box 6.3 conforming to legislation, does not either a) identify contingent problems of the kind described here or b) afford solutions to such problems. Nor is it inherent in the skills or competencies of any business that they should necessarily understand how to identify and resolve such problems and thereby manage change.

## Specialism as a barrier to change

The very qualities that lead to successful operation within an organisation and which were refined and enhanced over the passage of time, optimised to promote excellence or quality, become not an asset but a hindrance in the context of a changed or changing organisation. There are three reasons:

- The skill base will have been focused by the demands of the old system(s); it is therefore likely not to meet all the demands of the new operating environment
- Having acquired and been rewarded for one set of skills and way of operating, it becomes all the more difficult to 'see' the necessity of abandoning such skills, authority and power as will have flowed from being effective in the earlier operating context of the organisation
- It is highly unlikely that the existence and potential of radical alternatives to current technologies and practices will be recognised because problems and solutions will be considered within a given frame of reference

Foster (1986) provides many examples of large organisations that endured catastrophic collapse because they did not recognise the

---

**Box 6.4**

Environmental changes often transform earlier adaptive specialisations into cruel traps. As a changing environment passes beyond the range of a gene pool narrowed and made less versatile by specialisation, it often forces the extinction of a whole species. (E S Dunn, quoted in Weick 1979).

nature of the changes in their operating environment – changes that invalidated almost overnight systems with administrative and technical skills honed to the highest degree.

The NHS is replete with adaptations which have been made over decades. They are, or rather were, highly successful in conferring status, power, money and self-respect upon the staff who shared that milieu. It would be a mistake to expect that they will either a) adjust rapidly (if at all) or b) see the sense of abandoning current practices. This analysis would suggest that change will be hard to achieve within the framework as it exists.

If this analysis is valid, that change will occur when the opportunity to make changes passes out from current structures. The switch of emphasis to primary care and GP fundholding as a source of initiatives in provision and care management will create an arena for initiative that did not previously exist.

## Difficulty in gaining the appropriate level of involvement

This can include difficulty in getting any cooperation, in terms of positive commitment, whatsoever. New managers may find it hard to elicit basic systems information and this can occur at a number of levels. A new manager may find it difficult to get a clear statement as to exactly how far s/he has authority over the recruitment of staff and setting of budgets, or, at the other end of the spectrum, even basic information about how tasks are carried out may be missing or difficult to collect.

The task of implementing change becomes harder for example, when nominees are sought for training courses, or when an increased workload during a changeover period causes delays and extra work. The actual behaviours of individuals are many and various, but the principle is the same: non-cooperation even in a relatively passive form is very hard to measure, but it can very easily slow down or halt a project.

---

**Activity 6.2**

Think of a change which has been implemented in your workplace.
　What tactics did you/your colleagues employ which helped or hindered the change process?

---

There are numerous reports of the very significant impact that not cooperating with management can have upon the process of introducing a new system. Meetings are cancelled or delayed, data is incomplete, missing or inappropriate, a shortage of time and staff resources means constant delay and can inhibit implementation of new work systems. Obviously there are many other strategies, but the possibilities of employees preventing or delaying the implementation of change are many.

## New system(s) poorly used or rejected entirely

This is a subcategory of the lack of cooperation issue, but it can be due to a failure in the design of the new procedures so it deserves some further attention.

Poor usage of the revised or new system can be seen to take a number of forms, all of which can be damaging to the long-term viability of the new business process. If particular facilities remain unused and performance suffers as a consequence, then it is clear that there has been a failure either to motivate or train staff appropriately. The difference, however, between a failure to train and a failure to motivate is important and should be identified so that appropriate remedial steps can be taken.

In either case the cost can be high, especially if the overall level of performance offers no advantage over earlier procedures or system(s). If such a situation persists, it will contribute to resistance to the system: failure feeds on itself and the 'honeymoon' period for new systems is unfortunately very short, especially when resistance develops before it is introduced. The benefits of new working practices have to become obvious very quickly to overcome initial hostility.

In the case of users employing the changed system in ways not provided for, or required by the designers, there can be a number of causes. First and perhaps most damning of all, is the situation where misuse occurs out of ignorance. In this situation overcomplex system design and/or inadequate training may be the cause.

## Apathy

A more problematic reason for such behaviour is the situation where users are apathetic about the new system. As a consequence little effort is made to use the system to the full. Apathy therefore predicts a very low level of system utilisation, probably linked to a preference for and perhaps even a preservation of the old working methods. An extreme manifestation of the 'withdrawal stage' of resistance is the total rejection of the systems. There is therefore a great deal of work to be done at a senior level in overcoming this serious problem. While it remains a question of apathy, repeated training efforts and close monitoring can redress the situation.

## Regression

As the problem deepens and facilities are misused this can indicate two types of user response: the first is the *regressive*, where the user will not attempt to acquire any new skills and is therefore perfectly capable of making errors that did not occur before. Thus the new system can be seen to create a class of problems that did not exist before its inception, a situation which makes progress that much harder. Regression means that a more positive action is required and the trainer can expect little response to her/his efforts. Certainly, no training aids based upon a degree of trainee motivation such as manuals, check lists, advice lines and query systems can function in such an atmosphere.

## Active rejection

The more contentious stage is where systems misuse forms part of an active rejection of the system. It is important that the scale of this activity is borne in mind. If large numbers of users are behaving in this fashion this should be considered as a symptom of a failure of the implementation process or the systems design. The question of how to deal with individuals who deliberately sabotage the system is a separate issue.

## Beating the system

It should also be remembered that behaviours that are an obvious malpractice to system designers may seem otherwise to users of the system. For example, strategies quickly occur for 'beating the system', creating short cuts through what appears to be excessively detailed and unnecessary procedures. This is a training fault. Users need to know what to do, but also why; they can then judge for themselves the impact of strategies that from ignorance may appear to be practical alternatives.

## Characteristic general rejection responses

We have already discussed some of the consequences of a user response, or lack of response, in the form of apathy. At this point it is useful to point out how deleterious such a response is in the long term. New and revised management systems or work practices require a considerable amount of maintenance. In the early months a host of problems occur, and require the cooperation of users both to identify and to remove. If no such positive contribution from the user population is forthcoming, the short-term productivity of a new system is threatened and its long-term viability is open to question.

There are many other reasons why a positive acceptance of new practices is required: for example, the morale of a user site can decline dramatically without it. The implementation process must therefore be based upon the need to establish an encouraging atmosphere, not simply on the desire to 'get it in' and see what happens. The consequences of inadequate preparation in terms of identifying user needs and abilities are as important as any technical constraints upon performance.

### Projection

Few of the characteristic responses mentioned here occur alone; they may characterise one level of the response within an organisation or simply one feature of a response made up of a loose and variable body of attitudes and positions. Nevertheless, a variety of responses exist and can be isolated in turn. Projection is a response which can often occur as part of a rejection syndrome. In this case, the system can become the focus for a large number of grievances not all of which are strictly related to the inception of a new system. In short, anything and everything which goes wrong will be blamed on the system.

This in turn leads to two sets of problems: on the one hand the problem or fault is seen to be the responsibility of someone else – 'them', 'those up there' and so on – but certainly not the concern of the users themselves. This means that there is no impetus for individuals or group users to do anything but criticise, i.e. it will not be constructive criticism nor will it necessarily reach the ears of those who might correct faults in the system. Thus the stage is set for the decline of system performance over a very short period.

The second problem is perhaps more serious and there is some indirect evidence that projection underlies a lot of friction caused by new systems. The change proposed becomes a symbol, a sticking point, one final issue where all grievances are aired. This is hardly surprising, as in many cases new systems have been designed and implemented that are in themselves a concentrated expression of all the inadequacies of non-management that complex organisations are capable of. This situation is to be avoided at all costs, but unfortunately it reflects the importance of the past record of a company, rather than its response to future changes. This is only relatively important in so far as an organisation views its own past record in these matters to be poor. Obviously this varies from one location to another, and some portents for the future may be gleaned from existing circumstances and recent history of a given location.

## INDIVIDUAL RESPONSES TO CHANGE

Individual responses to changes in the circumstances and content of work are highly variable, compounded even more because it is very difficult to isolate responses that are the consequence of change from those responses that are a direct result of having to use new technology as part of the change.

There are a large number of physical reactions that the circumstances of change can bring about. The disruption and uncertainty that can characterise the period of transition have been known to induce such reactions as headaches, nausea, demotivation and listlessness. A general change in the tempo of work and the 'atmosphere' of the workplace, which is almost entirely negative in its consequences, can result.

The increased rate of illness during the period of change is often a genuine reduction in the physical well-being of staff and not necessarily an attempt to avoid the increased workload and other difficult conditions of a period of transition. In short, it is difficult to avoid the conclusion that the process of change can be highly stressful for many of those affected.

An increase in absenteeism is obviously going to be associated with such physical disorders, but can also reflect a loss of commitment and general lack of interest. This means that upsets that would not have previously kept an employee away from work will now be sufficient reason not to attend. These characteristic responses may converge on the one strategy – resignation.

**Box 6.5**  Range of possible attitudes to change

1. **Positive support** manifest in active contributions to implementing and developing new practices
2. **Widespread acceptance.** This reduces the need to use sanctions but suggests that little contribution can be expected to emerge from the workforce beyond their acceptance
3. **A cooperative response.** This requires control and direction from above and implies a need for thorough control – i.e. detailed direction that may not have been required before and may not be available during the period of transition
4. **A passive response.** This can be dysfunctional in so far as feedback from employees on the problems or failings of the new practices will not be given
5. **Apathy.** As well as leading to an unfortunate work atmosphere, this certainly involves long-term problems for the manager/supervisor and a reduction in the benefits to be derived from the new approach, whatever it might be
6. **Regressive response.** Employees will not actively learn from experience with the new approach; performance will not improve with experience and the new practises will take longer to 'bed in'; there will be a tendency to cling to the old ways of doing things
7. **Withdrawal.** A passive form of resistance, this response will have strongly negative effects and creates difficulties for managers, supervisors and training staff
8. **Protests.** The beginnings of active opposition; as well as indicating immediate and local problems for management this type of response can spread quickly within and between units – perhaps the most significant problem is the difficulty of overcoming such a response while the new system is still being operationalised
9. **Deliberate sabotage.** Anyone who can manipulate a system to her/his own ends can begin to do damage

An increase in labour turnover – the rate at which staff leave and a decrease in the period of time they spend with the company – is another symptom. When an employee cannot leave, because of pressing circumstances such as financial obligations and a job shortage, then the frustration will probably further reduce efficiency even though the company has been spared some of the costs associated with a high attrition rate.

Responses nos 1–5 in Box 6.5 are stages (acceptance to indifference) that can be tolerated, although it is unlikely that apathy can be overcome by force, so the system(s) will never operate optimally. Responses nos 6–9 are costly and imply loss of efficiency which could well prove to be a permanent feature of the new system(s) and those charged with operating them. These stages of active rejection imply a considerable failure, even if the situation is resolved and strongly suggest the need for a review of the way in which planning and managing change was undertaken.

---

**Activity 6.3**

Identify a possible change which could cause conflict within your own work situation. Consider the likely reactions of the staff towards that change. Describe the positive and negative behaviours that could result.

---

## THE PSYCHOLOGICAL CONTRACT

Many of the issues discussed above have been brought into focus by the concept of the psychological contract (Rousseau 1989). This concept can be used to frame our understanding of the exchange relationship between employer and employee. Simply put, the psychological contract is conceptualised as a sophisticated set of expectations and rules which forms the psychological basis for the continuing commitment of employees to their employers. More recently researchers have sought to identify how many different forms of contract there may be and how they are formed (Shore & Tetrick 1994). It would appear from studies of the concept that it does indeed have considerable explanatory power, not least when it comes to the question of explaining what it is that employers have to lose when organisational change can cause the breakdown of such contracts (Guzzo et al 1994).

The psychological contract can be understood as a system of expectations the employee forms concerning what the employer should be offering – should the employer offer job security, for example? Also included are expectations placed upon the employee by the employer, for instance that employees should place the company's needs before those of their family during working hours. Both sets of expectations help to form the contract. Similarly, both parties have beliefs about what the other party expects; so, for example, my employer knows that I expect a degree of job security – whether or not my employer believes that I *should* expect it. Finally, it would appear that as well as beliefs and expectations both parties have views as to what is actually the case in any given employer–employee relationship – e.g. how much job security do I actually have? Rousseau (1989) suggests that the psychological contract is a highly personal, subjective notion which governs the behaviour of the employee towards the employers as it develops over time.

## Transactional versus relational contracts

The relevance of all this for the current discussion of change derives from the view that these expectations lead to two different kinds of contract. The first kind, known as transactional (Parks 1992) is based on the economic obligation placed upon an employer when the employee produces effective work. This is an economic transaction between two parties resolved entirely in terms of the work carried out and the economic reward that ensues. On the other hand, a relational obligation is a form of contract in which social rather than economic exchange is the focus (Shore & Tetrick 1994). The contract based upon social exchange contains unspecified obligations that are not formalised into the contract of employment and the fulfilment of these expectations is thereby based on trust, not formal obligation (Blau 1964). Just because the relational contract covers areas not set out in formal terms does not make the expectations of the two parties any the less serious or important for the business; because issues such as trust, obligation and commitment cannot be given an unambiguous price they are frequently based on a relational obligation that reflects their considerable importance to the business and individual employee. Some aspects of the relational contract can be assigned a monetary value, but such valuations largely do not cover personal, socioemotional and value-based expectations of employees and employers. For example, contracts can be designed to retain some members of staff for a fixed period; the psychological contract developed over many years of loyal service is not discharged by the simple monetary compensation offered on redundancy or demotion.

The importance of the relational contract derives in part from the behaviours that are felt to be governed by this type of contract. As already discussed, these are the areas characterised by ambiguity and personal judgements. The extra-role or citizenship behaviours are perhaps the most relevant in a discussion of change. Briefly, it has been argued (Parks 1992) that the contributions that employees make to the organisation over and above that which might be expected, including looking out for opportunities to serve the company and putting the company's interests before their own, are the fruits of a relational contract. Perhaps the key function of the psychological contract in the context of change and much of what has been written above about employee reactions to change is that because of the contract the individual employee will monitor his or her own behaviour. Because of the perceived nature of the psychological contract between employer and employee, the employee will seek to meet the contract in terms of actions not specified in terms of the formal contract of employment but essential to the successful management of change. In other words, in the absence of direct orders from a supervisor the employee will discharge a perceived moral obligation to serve the best interests of the company. As we have already seen change produces a variety of unintended consequences; obviously the commitment of employees to act for the best, whether or not they have been ordered to do so, is a major asset in the bid to 'manage' change.

---

**Activity 6.4**

As an employee of the NHS, can you list the obligations you must fulfil ('extra-role behaviours') which are not specified in your contract of employment?

---

By the same token, the consequence of violating the psychological contract will be to impose unpredictable but real costs on the process of change management. As a result of violating the psychological contract the individual can give voice to his or her feelings in order to restore the contract, simply be silent, retreat and/or exit from the situation (Shore & Tetrick 1994). As can be seen, this maps very well on to the typology of individual change reactions described above. In the main, violations of transactional contracts are short-term in their effects but relational contracts based on mutual trust can only be violated with more serious and long-term consequences. In fact, Rousseau (1989) describes intense responses such as anger and moral outrage as the response to violation of relational contracts. This is particularly the case if the employee attributes the responsibility for the violation to the organisation rather than external forces.

The role of the psychological contract is to allow the individual to make sense of the experience of work and to maintain or develop a model of his or her relationship with the employer over time. The contract tells the employee who they are, what they are doing and why they are doing it. It takes time to develop such a contract and time to change it. It is perfectly possible to manage staff in such a way as to deny the existence of such 'informal' psychological bonds between the employing organisation and its employees. The psychological contract is nonetheless a reality and its implications for the efficiency of organisations, particularly when it is denied or ignored, are more difficult to set aside.

## CONCLUSION

In order to manage change we need a practical theory as to what change actually is. Change is a *continuous process* and cannot be understood or managed from the point of view of dealing with a discrete event or a particular group of changes. Change interventions designed to manage or promote change that do not incorporate this notion of a continuous process will not serve complex organisations. Following on from this it is possible to suggest that adequate change never occurs on time and is never 'over', because it cannot occur either on schedule or before it is needed in many cases. It follows therefore than an organisation is best prepared for change by always being capable of changing; either by constantly producing new ideas or by being able to recognise and exploiting ideas originated elsewhere. Also, unless the business is capable of a high level of reflexive awareness, i.e. understands itself and its operating environment, it will find it difficult to act in time to survive major changes in its environment. The normal focus of management attention and indeed the importance of 'doing' rather than reflecting in management culture generally, militates against the degree of organisational self-awareness that is required for managing change.

This is the greatest threat in an age of change; to continue as before in order to create and meet goals as yet unanticipated is to invite failure. To deal with each experience of change as though it were an objective fact – 'we must do something about X' – is to miss the point. Each event is a product of a complex system of constraints acting between individuals, groups, the organisation and its environment. It is only by acting in terms of this model that we can hope to manage change processes rather than exist within them.

Preplanned and problem-focused change and change management cannot be the sole answer to an organisation's need to change. Culture and organisational interventions such as selection procedures, team building strategies, reward systems, alternative management structures – even dress codes and attendance requirements – need to be looked at. Clearly, change management interventions that concentrate on the structure of an organisation while neglecting the culture will be inadequate. Change management cannot be entirely rational, planned in advance or based solely on empirical data and analysis. Consequently the short-term, problem-focused approach to managing change is a myth: this approach to the problem is not effective management nor does it foster or 'control' the impact of change.

---

**Activity 6.5**

Using the definitions given within this chapter, how would you differentiate between the two concepts of change and innovation and what is their relationship?

---

REFERENCES

Anderson N (1992) Work group innovation: a state of the art review. In Hosking I D M, Anderson N (ed) Organisational change and innovation, psychological perspectives and practices in Europe. Routledge, London

Anderson B, Ginnerup L (1992) The support of cognitive capacity in future organisations: towards enhanced communicative competence and cooperative problem-structuring capability. In Rasmussen, JHB Anderson, NO Bernson (ed) Human computer interaction: research directions in cognitive science: European perspectives, vol.3. Lawrence Erlbaum Associates, Hove

Blackler F (1992) Formative contexts and activity systems: postmodern approaches to the management of change. In Reed M, Hughes M (eds) Rethinking organization: new directions in organization theory and analysis. Sage, London, pp 273-294

Blau P M (1964) Exchange and power in social life. John Wiley, New York

Brunsson N (1985) The irrational organisation. John Wiley, Chichester

Caines E (1994) The impact of trusts on the management of the NHS. Health Services Management Research 7(3): 181-183

Cartwright S, Cooper C L (1994) The human effects of mergers and acquisitions. In Cooper C L, Rousseau D M (ed) Trends in organisational behaviour, vol 1. John Wiley, Chichester

Daft R L (1982) Bureaucratic verses non-bureaucratic structure and the process of innovation and change. In Bacharach S B (ed) Research in the sociology of organisations. JAI Press, Greenwich, C T

Damanpour F (1990) Innovation, effectiveness, adoption and organisational performance. In West M A, Farr J (ed) Innovation and creativity at work. John Wiley, Chichester

Eason K (1988) Information technology and organisational change. Taylor & Francis, London

Foster R (1986) Innovation: the attacker's advantage. Macmillan, London

Guzzo R A, Noonan K A, Elron E (1994) Expatriate managers and psychological contract. J Appl Psycol 79(4): 617–626

Haggard P (1993) I think therefore I manage. Health Service J: 26–27

Hales C (1993) Managing through organisation. Routledge, London

Hosking D M, Anderson N (1992) Organisational change and innovation: psychological perspectives and practices in Europe. Routledge, London

Kritzman L D (1988) Politics, philosophy, culture: interviews and other writings, 1977–1984. Routledge, London

McKeown M (1995) The transformation of nurses' work? J Nurs Management 3: 67–73

Nicholson N (1990) Organisational innovation in context. In West M, Farr J Innovation and creativity at work. John Wiley, Chichester

Nystrom H (1990) Organisational innovation. In West M, Farr J Innovation and creativity at work. John Wiley, Chichester

Parks J M (1992) The role of incomplete contracts and their role in the governance of delinquency, in-role and extra-role behaviours. Paper presented at the Society for Industrial and Organisational Psychology, Montreal

Peters J (1989) Thriving on chaos. Pan, London

Peters J (1992) Liberation management. Macmillan, London

Ranson S (1994) Towards a learning society. Cassell, London

Rousseau D M (1989) Psychological and implied contracts in organisations. Employee Responsibilities Rights J 2: 121–139

Salaman G, Butler J (1990) Why managers won't learn. Management Educ Devel 21(3): 183–191

Senge P M (1990) The fifth discipline: the art and practice of the learning organisation. Century Business, London

Shore L M, Tetrick L E (1994) The psychological contract as an exploratory framework in employment relationships. In Cooper CL, Rousseau DM (ed) Trends in organisational behaviour, vol 1. John Wiley, Chichester

Singleton W T (1989) The mind at work. Cambridge University Press, Cambridge

Spurgeon P, Barwell F (1991) Implementing change in the NHS: a practical guide for managers. Chapman & Hall, London

Weick C (1979) The social psychology of organising. Addison-Wesley, Reading, MA

West M A, Farr J (1990) Innovation and creativity at work. John Wiley, Chichester

Willcocks L, Mason D (1987) Computerising work: people, systems design and workplace relations. Paradigm Press, London

# Financing the National Health Service: a financial director's perspective

R. Dredge

## COST OF THE NATIONAL HEALTH SERVICE (NHS)

The NHS is one of the largest areas of Government spending. In 1994/95 it was planned that nearly £40 billion would be spent on the NHS in the UK. Table 7.1 analyses the components of expenditure.

The largest element – 73% – goes on the hospital, community health and Family Health Service Authority (FHSA) cash-limited services. This latter element covers areas such as the payment of GPs' practice staff and rental for premises. The 1.4% spent on

**Table 7.1** UK NHS spending 1994/95 (gross) (Department of Health Departmental Report, March 1994)

|  | £m | % |
|---|---|---|
| 1. NHS hospital, community, FHSA – cash limited | 28 711 | 73.0 |
| 2. NHS Trusts | 563 | 1.4 |
| 3. FHSA non-cash-limited | 8680 | 22.1 |
| 4. Departmental administration | 314 | 0.8 |
| 5. Central and miscellaneous services | 1042 | 2.7 |
| Total | 39 310 | 100.0 |

**Table 7.2** Source of funds (%) (Departmental Report, March 1994: CM 2521)

| Year | Treasury | Charges | Other |
|------|----------|---------|-------|
| 1989/90 | 94.1 | 4.5 | 1.4 |
| 1990/91 | 94.4 | 4.5 | 1.1 |
| 1991/92 | 94.9 | 4.1 | 1.0 |
| 1992/93 | 95.7 | 3.7 | 0.6 |
| 1993/94 | 95.7 | 3.5 | 0.8 |

trusts represents their set-up and running costs. Non-cash-limited FHSA expenditure comprises the 'demand-led' services such as drugs and dental services. While there is no apparent limit to the demand that can be met, there is still an overall budget set at national level. Departmental administration costs are those associated with the Department of Health itself. Central and other costs cover the NHS Executive, regional management executive offices, special health authorities and supraregional services. In addition to this £39 310 million, a further £1600 million is spent on capital items.

Health care in the UK is funded largely from public revenues. Services are largely free at the point of delivery and the contribution of charges to the total funding of the NHS has declined in recent years. Table 7.2 shows the sources of funding of the NHS and the recent trends in their contribution.

Charges are predominantly those associated with primary care services such as prescriptions, dental and ophthalmic test fees. Other income is mainly that from capital receipts arising from the sale of surplus land. The contribution from the Treasury is paid for through the collection of taxes. All revenue received by the Treasury is held in a single fund – the Consolidated Fund. Payments to Government spending programmes come from this fund. There are no taxes guaranteed or earmarked as being specifically for any programme such as health.

The NHS has enjoyed a consistent increase in funding in recent years. For the 3 years to 1994/95 this averaged 2.2% a year over and above the rate of inflation.

---

**Activity 7.1**

Look again at Table 7.2. Note that the contribution to NHS funding from charges such as fees for eye tests and dental check-ups has diminished since 1989/90 by 1%.
What could account for this reduction in income from direct charges?

---

## ALLOCATION OF FUNDS

Each year the Department of Health submits a bid to the Treasury for the funding of the NHS. These requests, along with those of all the other Government departments are reviewed in a process known as the Public Expenditure Survey Committee (PESC).

This process determines the overall affordability of all Government spending proposals. In so doing it takes account of the ability of the Government to fund the programme, the burden this places on the taxpayer and how much borrowing would be needed to bridge any shortfall between tax revenues and total planned spend. This sum is the public sector borrowing requirement (PSBR) and is a key tool in the Government's overall economic policy.

The PESC process is finalised in the presentation to Parliament of the Government's budget and spending plans. This happens in November of each year when the Chancellor of the Exchequer sets out his proposals for both spending and funding, through taxation, of the coming year's budgets. Parliament agrees these plans and then 'votes' allocations to specific programmes. Once a sum has been 'voted' to a programme by Parliament it cannot be used for any other purpose. There are, however, opportunities to add to, or change 'votes' in the twice-yearly spring and autumn estimates. These, in effect, are minor variations to plans to allow for changed circumstances.

---

**Activity 7.2**

Think back to the last budget and the Chancellor's autumn statement. How did Government raise income from taxation in order to fund total public expenditure?

---

The monies available to the NHS are, therefore, agreed by Parliament and allocated (voted) to the Department of Health. The

Department then has a duty to spend them for the purpose agreed by Parliament.

The Department of Health allocates funds to the purchasers of health care. Up until 1996 the process was that each regional health authority in England (Scotland, Wales and Northern Ireland being funded through their respective state offices) was allocated funds. They, in turn allocated to DHA/FHSA purchasers. From 1996 the Department of Health will allocate funds directly to purchasers, thus eliminating the role of the regional health authorities in financial allocations.

The method upon which allocations are made is that of 'weighted capitation'. This has been the case since 1976, when the basic principles of attempting to allocate resources that reflected an equitable share of the total available, based upon health needs, were first introduced. This process established the concepts of a target allocation – the allocation that a population should have on a fair-share basis, the fair share being in relation to the total planned spend on health. It does not take any direct account of the needs or demands for health care. The mechanics of establishing a target allocation and comparing the distance from target, can be explained by the simple example given in Table 7.3.

The total available resource (£200m) is to be allocated not on the historical 'current' basis, but on the equitable share of total population. The resource available is therefore split pro rata to population to give the target allocation. The distance from target is then easily calculated.

It has generally been the case that allocations have been 'evened up'. That is to say that over-target purchasers have rarely had allocations reduced, but under target purchasers have had extra monies, i.e. the annual growth allocation, given to them.

**Table 7.3** Allocation targets

| DHA | Population | Current allocation | Target allocation | Distance | % |
|---|---|---|---|---|---|
| | 000s | £m | £m | £m | |
| 1 | 500 | 110 | 100 | +10 | +10 |
| 2 | 250 | 40 | 50 | −10 | −20 |
| 3 | 250 | 50 | 50 | — | — |
| | 1000 | 200 | 200 | — | — |

**Table 7.4** Allocation of growth

| DHA | Current allocation £m | Revised allocation £m | Revised target allocation £m | Distance £m | % |
|---|---|---|---|---|---|
| 1 | 110 | 110 | 102 | +8 | +8 |
| 2 | 40 | 43 | 51 | –8 | –16 |
| 3 | 50 | 51 | 51 | — | — |
| | 200 | 204 | 204 | — | — |

In the above example let us say that there was a growth addition of 2% agreed as part of the annual PESC settlement. This would give £4 million (2% of £200m) as growth for the population. In order to ensure that the 'on-target' purchaser (DHA 3) does not fall below the average it must receive 2%, i.e. £1 million; the over-target purchaser should receive nothing and the balance of £3 million should go to the below-target purchaser. The position after the new allocation is illustrated in Table 7.4.

Note that the target has to be increased by the overall increased percentage to maintain a benchmark for a 'fair share'.

The differential allocation to purchasers, based on distance from target, will therefore bring all purchasers to their target. This process assumes a constant element of growth available to the NHS.

In 1995 the NHS Executive concluded a review of the actual funding formula to be used in this process. To reflect the perception of different health needs based upon socioeconomic and geographical factors certain indicators of need have been refined and included in the formula. The original research work was undertaken by York University. The NHS Executive has refined their findings to produce a more 'acceptable' model. Needs – based largely on morbidity – have always been used, but research has shown that a more robust assessment can be made if the following are included when considering general and acute services:

1. Standardised mortality ratio for age under 75: a proxy measure for morbidity
2. % unemployed
3. % pensioners living alone
   % in single-carer household

   } socioeconomic indicators of deprivation/needs

and so each factor is weighted into a formula based upon the resident population for all RHA and DHAs. This gives the 'weighted capitation' calculation. Two further elements are added to the formula. The population is weighted by age group to allow for the different costs of providing care that is dependent upon age (the age–cost curve). An adjustment for labour costs, to reflect broadly the extra costs of wages in the south-east, is also added in. The formula is explained in detail in the NHS Executive publication entitled *HCHS Review – Resource Allocation – Weighted Capitation Formula*.

---

**Activity 7.3**

Reflect on the socioeconomic factors that adversely affect the health of the local population in your own town. Which of these factors ought to lead, in your view, to the allocation of additional NHS resources to purchasers?

---

Currently RHAs can use their own formula, which may change the relativities of weighting. From 1996/97 a standard national formula will be used. This will be seen to be objective and transparent. It will remove any accusation of special treatment for any specific purchaser or patient group.

The growth additions described above are for funds over and above those needed to maintain the existing services – 'the baseline'. The cost of this increases every year as a result of the import of inflation (pay and price rises). The PESC settlement allows for this by adding an across-the-board figure to all allocations. This is the Government's assessment of the cost (rate) of inflation.

## INCOME – PROVIDERS OF HEALTH SERVICES

Providers are not funded on any formula, but simply earn the income that arises from work done. This is predominantly from patient care contracts and extracontractual referrals. The total income of a provider, e.g. an NHS trust, is wholly dependent upon the ability to persuade purchasers of the need for the services and to ensure that they pay for them.

Providers will have many sources of income, each with an associated degree of risk of it being collected. A system of contracting has

**Table 7.5** Purchasing by risk type – % spend (Health Database, CIPFA/ HFMA 1992, 1993, 1994)

| Income type | 1992/93 | 1993/94 | 1994/95 |
|---|---|---|---|
| Category A: Patient services, fixed at start of year | 97.8 | 96.9 | 93.5 |
| Category B: Patient services, varies with activity | 1.4 | 2.4 | 4.5 |
| Category C: Other | 0.8 | 0.7 | 2.0 |

developed whereby a provider will agree with any purchaser to provide a given volume of health care to a given quality for a given price. This means that providers have to manage the income flow from a large number of sources and ensure that they all add up to cover the expenditure being incurred to provide these services.

In financial planning terms the risk associated with each type of contract is:

- *Block contract*: financially risk free; income guaranteed
- *Cost and volume*: relatively risk-free; large element guaranteed; 'volume' element generally at marginal cost, so directly related to work done
- *Cost per case*: high risk, as no guarantee of income

The most comfortable financial position is one with the least at-risk income. This is because annual expenditure budgets will be set on the assumption of a mix of types of contract income. Once a budget is set and resources committed the income must be generated to cover expenditure. If at-risk income does not materialise – e.g. one assumes 100 referrals at a cost-per-case payment, but only 50 actually arise – then the income gap has to be met by reduced expenditure.

1994/95 was the fourth year of the NHS internal market. The extent to which risk has been extended through contracts being based directly on the volume of patient services provided is shown by Table 7.5. This demonstrates the way purchasers have contracted and intend to contract with their allocations. There is a small movement away from the no-risk Category-A-type income. As the market develops then it can be expected that this trend will continue and probably escalate.

**Activity 7.4**

Re-read the 'Income-providers of health services' paragraphs again. Note that a 'block contract' brings with it guaranteed income to the provider; hence it is 'low-risk' in financial terms.

From Table 7.5, note that in 1992/3 97.8% of purchasing was in block contracts, compared to 93.5% in 1994/5. Hence, guaranteed income to providers is less secure now than it was in 1992/3, i.e. they face more risk of income not matching expenditure requirements.

## COSTING AND PRICE REGULATIONS

The introduction of the internal market was designed, partly, to release the spirit of enterprise, innovation and change that comes with competition. However, hospitals in the NHS could not be allowed to compete on price alone. If they did the risk was that, quickly, one hospital could put out of business a neighbouring hospital. The Government did not want to see this happen, as a basic underlying aim of the NHS is appropriate access to local care. Instead, the internal market was introduced with a range of market regulations, rules and controls in order to increase performance while obtaining maximum value for money.

The fundamental rules of costing and pricing are that:

- Price equals cost
- Cost is based upon the full average cost of the service
- There is no planned cross subsidisation

Prices are subject to independent audit to ensure that these rules are applied.

In themselves these rules are eminently sensible, in the context of the NHS. They should ensure that:

- No profit or surplus is made or at least planned to be made. A surplus for a provider implies that money has been taken from purchasers that was not needed to cover the cost of services provided. That money could otherwise have been used to purchase more work
- Competition is at true cost, and thus relative efficiency and inefficiency, in cost terms, becomes apparent to both purchasers and providers. The market would then decide if these were to be tolerated or if pressure should be applied to improve cost performance

- All purchasers are treated equally in price terms, i.e. everyone is charged the same

While these rules have been applied generally and broadly, there is evidence that there has not been universal application.

These rules apply to the once-a-year setting of prices. The system operates on an annual contracting round that comes together in March in readiness for the new financial year commencing on 1 April.

## COST STRUCTURES

NHS providers are required to classify costs in a standardised and uniform way. This ensures that cost and (because cost equals price) price comparisons are made on a consistent basis. Any differences are not due to variations in accounting treatment.

There are two elements to the understanding of costs. These are the type of cost and its behaviour. Cost types are categorised as being one of:

- *Direct cost*: can be attributed directly to the activity or outputs being measured; includes items such as drugs, ward staff, direct treatment costs
- *Indirect cost*: shared over a number of facilities; apportioned or allocated depending on the amount used; include catering, linen and laundry, teaching programmes
- *Overhead*: cost of support services contributing to the general running of the hospital, but not directly related to services provided by specific departments

| Activity 7.5 |
| --- |
| Think of the running costs associated with a large general hospital of 800 beds. Which services could be counted as general overheads? (One example to get you started – general management.) |

These cost types may be treated differently by different providers. The test is how costs are managed and accounted for. For example, if there is a conventional central portering service that responds to requests across all services provided, it is an overhead. If there are dedicated porters in a department they can be seen as a direct cost.

The second element in understanding costs is to appreciate cost behaviour. That is how a cost changes with a change in activity. The usual way of categorising these is as follows:

- *Fixed*: unaffected by activity in a 1-year period, e.g. rates, service agreements for equipment
- *Semi-fixed*: fixed for a given amount of activity, but may rise or fall as activity changes; also called step costs ('once and for all costs'), these include most staff costs
- *Variable*: costs that change in relation to activity; e.g. drugs and laboratory consumables

These definitions refer to behaviour over the normal operating range – the level of activity planned for the facility.

Cost behaviour and in particular the importance of understanding where changes in cost occur can be presented as in Figure 7.1. Fixed costs remain constant irrespective of activity; semi-fixed cost steps are represented by the once-and-for-all increase in costs. Variable costs are shown through the slope of the cost line between the semi-fixed cost points. An example of why this knowledge is important for both purchasers and providers can be taken from Figure 7.1. Assume that a purchaser wishes to increase the number of cases bought by 5%. If

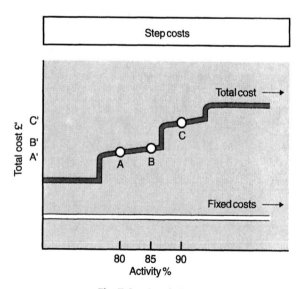

**Fig 7.1** Cost behaviour

the provider is operating at 80% of capacity and moves to the 85% position, a cost increase of B minus A is incurred. This reflects only the variable cost. If, however, a further move of 5% is desired from 85% to 90% of capacity, a cost change of C minus B is incurred. This includes a step cost, e.g. a new consultant or staffing for more beds. The cost shift C – B is clearly more than B – A. However, note that more work can be undertaken beyond point C, at variable cost only.

---

**Activity 7.6**

- Refer again to Figure 7.1
- Note the cost A' of providing 80% activity (say £200 000)
- Note that increasing activity to 85% will result in costs rising to B' (say £220 000)
- Therefore the 5% increase in activity has resulted in increased costs of £20 000
- These are *variable* costs associated with variations in activity
- Note that to shift another 5%, to 90% activity, leads to costs rising to C' (say £300 000), or £80 000 for a 5% increase in workload
- These 'step costs' arise because a critical point has been reached whereby major expenditure is needed to cope with the total activity, e.g. one additional consultant

---

## SETTING THE PRICE

In order to establish the price at which to agree contracts or to undertake work, a full knowledge of the costs incurred in the provision of the service is required. This is not only because price must recover cost, but because cost is equal to price in the NHS. Therefore, setting the cost is the same as setting the price.

There are two approaches that can be used. They are termed 'top-down', which takes the total cost of running the service and ensures it is allocated in full, and 'bottom-up', which relies on costing of the inputs and resources needed to provide the service.

The 'top-down' method is a 'desktop' approach. The stages, for an acute provider, are:

1. Identify the provider-wide total cost that you expect to incur in the financial year, based upon your inputs, resource utilisation and expected level of work, and any retention agreed in your business plan

2. Next, at Stage 2, you have to classify the costs on the basis of the national standards. This then allows you to

3. Allocate and apportion to patient treatment services. At the end of this you have allocated all your overheads and non-patient costs to clinical areas. At this stage you can slice costs for an average FCE in a speciality. This becomes your price, and total activity × price = cost of service

4. Finally, you must reconcile to your provider-wide total cost because price × volume gives you operating income, which has to cover operating costs

This process is described in a simplified way in Figure 7.2.

Increasingly, costing is being approached 'from the bottom up' (Fig. 7.3). This involves the following steps and is based on a speciality-by-speciality approach.

1. Identify the actual activity undertaken by procedure-specific groups such as health-related groups (HRGs). These can be thought of as the 'product lines' of the specialty

2. Agree, through interviews with clinicians, which procedures from the HRG analysis take up most of their resources. This step is necessary to check and clarify the accuracy of clinical coding

3. Define clearly which HRG and/or procedure to cost

4. Agree cost profiles for each of these procedures and produce a 'bill of quantities' – a schedule of the inputs that go into the average case

5. Value the cost profile by costing each of the inputs adding to a total procedure cost

6. By multiplying the cost (= price) by the value of each procedure and adding for the whole specialty you will get the total specialty cost. This must be compared to the control total for the specialty obtained from a top-down or budget approach. This reconciliation is vital, because the final price will be used to give the income required to cover the cost of producing the work

7. Lastly, review and agree the prices to ensure that clinicians and their teams understand them

The pricing process described above should be considered alongside the anticipated expenditure. If followed it means that at the start of a

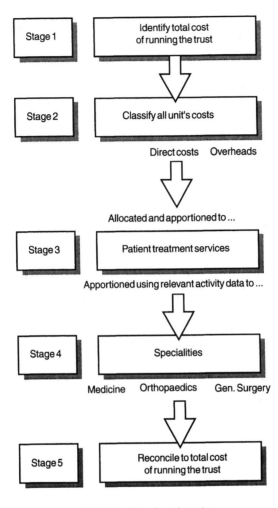

**Fig 7.2** 'Top-down' costing

financial year all expected costs are planned to be received through the income from contracts. In particular it means that:

- All fixed costs will be recovered
- All semi-fixed costs within the normal operating range have been recovered
- Variable costs incurred in providing the planned activity level are recovered

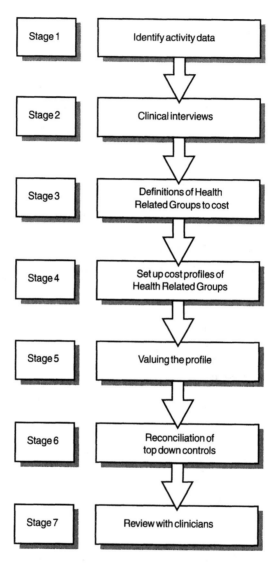

**Fig 7.3** 'Bottom-up' costing

This has interesting connotations for the rest of the financial year because if the price = cost rule is applied any additional new work can be taken on at variable cost only. This gives a clear incentive to purchasers to hold back from writing contracts until after 1 April, because those who have committed before 1 April have done so at full average cost on an assumed level of output for the hospital. Any new work needs only to recover variable costs and any step in semi-fixed costs.

Marginal cost contracts can only be agreed and sustained in the financial year they are agreed. Under the price = cost rules the new level of activity and costs will be shared under the pricing rules described earlier. This means, other things being equal, that while average costs will fall the total bill to any purchaser may rise. The marginal cost work has been replaced by work at a new full average cost.

## FINANCIAL CONTROL

All NHS organisations have a duty to ensure that their annual budget is not overspent. This operates at two levels:

- *Cash limits*: Purchasers are allocated a cash allocation, the fixed sum that they can draw from the Treasury in the course of a year. It cannot be exceeded no matter what the perceived health needs of the local population may be
- *Income and expenditure*: Providers will work to an income budget estimated from the total value of contracts and from the anticipated non-contract income. Expenditure must be contained within that total

Cash and income and expenditure accounting are different. Cash is simply the total cash available and spent. It is accounted for as and when it is dispersed, irrespective of purpose. Income and expenditure and cash differences are related to the timing of the use of the money. An example (Box 7.1) will explain.

---

**Box 7.1**

---

Assume there is a maintenance agreement for a piece of equipment that costs £10 000 for a 12-month period, and that it is payable in advance on 30 September. Financial years, in the NHS, run from 1 April to 31 March. This payment falls exactly halfway through the financial year. In accounting terms the treatment is:

- **Cash:** Paid on 30 September, Year 1; charge £10 000 cash account for that year
- **Income and expenditure:** As the expenditure covers financial years the charge is equal for each 6 months, i.e. £5000 in Year 1 and £5000 in Year 2.

Providers will work to an income budget estimated from the total value of contract and anticipated non-contract income. Expenditure must be contained within that total.

In overall terms both cash and income and expenditure targets have to be met.

Financial control is examined, generally, at two levels in the organisation. This is at the executive (Board) level and at the level of line managers. The Board level will need to be assured that key financial targets are being met. This will require them to have regular, timely and accurate financial information. These should contain details of the planned, actual and year-end projected position on cash and overall income and expenditure. The Board will reserve a right to instigate corrective action if variances arise that could result in the failure to meet targets.

The Director of Finance is required to submit periodic returns to the NHS Executive that give a clear picture of the organisation's financial position. These are generally produced at the end of each quarter (i.e. four times a year). If the organisation has a financial problem, the Executive can require monthly, and in exceptional cases weekly, monitoring returns. In addition to this control the NHS Executive requires that the Director of Finance informs her/his Board, on a monthly basis, of:

- The actual, budget and variance figures for the month
- The actual, budget and variance figures for the year to date
- The forecast budget and variance figures for the full year

The Board should receive reports that show information on the reasons for variances, and in particular contract performance, and will

---

**Box 7.2**

Trust Boards must:

- Ensure that they do not exceed their external financing limit (EFL)
- Ensure that expenditure does not exceed income
- Ensure that there is a 6% return on the value of net assets (the average of assets owned at the start of the year and the end of the year)

These are further described in the section on 'Financial duties', below.

---

**Box 7.3**

---

The external financing limit is how much additional money the Trust needs to carry out its business plan, primarily financing such things as 'one-off' capital costs.

---

require the Director of Finance to establish procedures of financial control. These will include internal checks, separation of duties and the production and monitoring of financial procedures. There will also be the need to provide an internal audit service that satisfies NHS minimum standards.

These measures indicate that financial control is exercised at the Executive and Board level and that systems of control are in place. However, for most managers the interest in the achievement of financial targets is likely to be at a more detailed level – that of the budgetary performance of those areas of the organisation for which they are responsible. If these are acceptable and all other managers are meeting their targets, it is reasonable to assume that the overall organisations targets will be met.

The directorate/departmental budget should be set on the basis that it funds, having due regard to efficiency and effectiveness, the resources needed to deliver the services expected of it. For clinical services this will be the planned level of workload agreed in contracts and added to by the assumed level of extracontractual work. For non-clinical services it will be the resources needed to support the clinical departments in their delivery of patient activity.

The expenditure budget becomes a plan of expenditure for the forthcoming year. The basis upon which it is set will vary from place to place. However, the key principles that should be used include:

- It must be based upon the resources needed to deliver the service required of the department. These will reflect the efficient use of resources and allow for the appropriate level of quality as well as volume of work
- It must be costed at current rates and a clear understanding must be reached as to how changes in prices are to be reflected in the budget
- It must be agreed with the manager responsible for its achievement

**Box 7.4**

| Pay | Manpower | £ | Non-pay | £ |
|---|---|---|---|---|
| Nurses | | | Dressings | x |
| – by grade | x | x | Disposable linen | x |
| – by speciality | x | x | Drugs | x |
| Doctors | | x | Uniforms | x |
| – by grade | x | x | Medical equipment | |
| – GPCAs | x | x | – disposable | x |
| – locum cover | x | x | – non-disposable | x |
| Clerical support | x | x | | |
| Total pay | x | x | Total non-pay | x |

A budget should not be imposed and cannot be managed unless full responsibility for spending decisions are given to the same manager.

The budget will contain an allocation for all of the areas of resources for which the manager is responsible. The detail will be agreed locally, but a typical budget for a ward could contain the items listed in Box 7.4.

Increasingly, budget responsibility is being devolved to the ward level. This enables ward managers to control their expenditure and more importantly to determine what they spend their budget on. There is a temptation to take the amount of detail contained in the reports to a very low level, e.g. to report on every type of catheter used. While this may be of interest it will add an unnecessary cost to the reporting process. It will generally be unnecessary to have a separate budget for an item costing less than £1000.

The key to successful budgetary control is to have timely and adequate reporting on the major areas of cost. This will enable the manager to exercise control over the budgets that s/he is responsible for. Budget reports should show, for each budget line, the following items:

1. Budget description
2. Annual budget
3. Budget for proportionate part of financial year (the annual budget divided into appropriate parts, which may or may not equal one-12th of the total, depending on the timing of planned spend)
4. Total expenditure to date

5. Budget and expenditure for the reporting period – normally a calendar month
6. Variances – over- or underspends – from the annual versus cumulative spend

From this information the manager will be able to establish where variances (i.e. movements from budgets) arise. It is the early attention to variance, and the pursuit of corrective action, that ensures successful budget management.

Over- or underspends can arise from two causes. These are:

- Price variance: The cost of resources required to deliver the service has not been correctly reflected in the budget
- Volume variance: The volume of work ultimately performed is different from that assumed when the budget was set

Price variances that arise from changes in cost will usually be subject to an organisation-wide policy on how such changes are managed. Prices can and do go up and down. Generally, changes in price, often referred to as inflation, are accommodated by increases in budget. The organisation, in its corporate budget, will have negotiated an 'inflation uplift' as part of its contract income. This will be kept in one of two ways:

- As a central reserve that will allocate monies to budgets as and when there is evidence of a change in prices
- As a departmental/directorate allocation, the initial reserve allocated to each department on a pro-rata basis. The department then manages this as part of its total budget

Whatever the process, there will be a fixed sum available across the organisation. If price increases exceed this, then there is a problem that has to be resolved.

The assessment of the price changes is relatively easy. For pay costs there are national and/or local pay awards that deal with the pay rates for each type and grade of staff. The budget will be based upon the

---

**Box 7.5** Hospital Price Index

This is an index of prices calculated nationally. Included are such things as drugs, disposable items and energy.

**Table 7.6** Variance – a problem?

| Contract | Variance | |
|---|---|---|
| | Adverse | Positive |
| Block | No | Yes |
| Cost-per-case | Yes | No |

staff grades employed and the numbers employed in each grade. A simple calculation will give the added cost of the pay award. For non-pay most NHS organisations rely upon the Hospital Price Index. This is an index of prices of commodity types such as drugs, medical disposables, provisions and energy. It is calculated nationally from NHS contract prices. This is published nationally and changes in the index are reflected in changes in budgets.

This process means that the real value of budgets should be constant and fair. Provided the base budget is correct there should be no price variances, because the budget is adjusted to reflect changed input prices.

Increases or decreases in the volume of work undertaken may or may not be a problem. If variance arises from a block contract, whereby less work is being undertaken (called an adverse variance), then the variable cost of that work is saved. If the volume is exceeded (a positive variance) then the variable cost is incurred with no additional income. If the variance is on a cost-per-case contract and there is extra work then this suggests extra income. If the variance shows that cost-per-case work is below target then fixed and semi-fixed costs are not being recovered. In very simple terms we can describe this as in Table 7.6.

This shows that the nature of the variance on cost recovery is the key to managing its effect – not whether it is positive or adverse.

---

**Activity 7.7**

- Recap Activity 7.6 and ensure that you understand 'variable costs'
- Note that if less work than planned is undertaken as part of a block contract, then variable costs are saved
- Note that if more work than planned is undertaken as part of a block contract, then no additional income will result
- When cost-per-case contracts vary, then extra income should result from additional workload

One area of budgetary control that can cause confusion is the cost of the employment of staff. Many managers fail to appreciate the extra cost over and above salary. In essence the cost of an individual is:

1. Basic salary, plus
2. Enhancements (e.g. overtime, duty payments, on-call), plus
3. Employee's superannuation contribution (4% for NHS schemes) plus
4. Employee's National Insurance (variable increase with salary for employees earning over £10 400 – 10.2%, to be reduced to 10.0% in 1997)

and so, as a minimum for an employee earning over £10 400 (in 1995/96) there is an additional 14.2% 'on cost' that the employer must pay. For employees earning less than this the percentage is slightly lower.

## FINANCIAL DUTIES

The purchaser/provider split has led to two very different sets of financial duties that the NHS organisations have to deliver. These reflect, broadly, the way in which they are funded as well as basic financial control.

The purchaser of health care – the district health authorities – are funded by a direct grant through the capitation funding formula. This is an annual cash allocation and the DHA must not spend, in cash terms, more than it is allocated in a financial year. It is its cash limit. In addition to this it must also balance on an income and expenditure basis, taking account of cash payments, income due and movements in working balances.

Providers such as trusts generate the money they need to spend to deliver services through income from purchasers. A trust does, like a DHA, have a duty to balance its income and expenditure on an annual basis.

In addition to these duties, a NHS trust is required to achieve two further targets:

- It must stay within its external financing limit (this is the net sum it is allowed to borrow each year)
- It must achieve a 6% return on the assets it employs; this is done by adding 6% of the cost of its assets to revenue prices

The trust generates money to repay the Treasury for the loans and interest on loans through achieving the 6% rate of return.

## CAPITAL

So far this chapter has dealt with the financial management of revenue, i.e. the income and expenditure that is used to provide day-on-day services that run the organisation. Investment is needed to replace, sustain or expand the organisation, and this is generally known as capital. In simple terms, capital is expenditure that will provide facilities or equipment for use beyond 1 year.

The NHS has adopted a specific definition of capital that puts some boundaries on this concept. In essence capital is:

- Expenditure on a resource with an expected life of more than 1 year, and
- Expenditure of £5000 (including VAT) or more on the asset or collection of assets that are functionally independent; this includes:
  - the purchase of land and premises
  - equipment, including vehicles
  - cost of staff engaged on capital works
  - schemes of initial provision, exterior or improvement, including demolition

Expenditure on maintaining capital assets in working order is charged to revenue. Computer software, irrespective of its cost, is generally not accounted for as capital. A full definition is contained in the NHS Executive's capital charges manual.

Expenditure on capital is almost entirely undertaken by NHS trusts. Little capital is needed by purchasers. Trusts gain access to capital for larger schemes through the acceptance by the regional office of the Management Executive of a business case for the expenditure. This lays out the details of the scheme, the costs of the capital outlay and the benefits that the scheme will bring. The benefits may be financial – revenue cost savings, for example, through rationalisation or a more revenue-efficient design. Equally, the service and quality benefits that the scheme brings will be assessed.

Smaller capital expenditure on minor items of equipment will be financed through an annual discretionary capital allocation. This is a lump sum that the trust can use in whatever way it sees fit, provided it is spent on capital items.

The level at which regional office approval is required depends on the size of the trust. Currently (1995/96) the limits are:

- Trust turnover up to £30 million – £250 000
- Trust turnover £30–80 million – £600 000
- Trust turnover over £80 million – £1 000 000

Schemes costing below the limit can be funded from discretionary capital. Hence a large trust has the power to spend £5000–1 000 000 on capital with no further approval needed.

All schemes over £10 million require the approval of the Treasury. The Treasury requires that all schemes irrespective of their costs, have examined the option of being funded by the private sector (the 'private finance initiative').

Before a business case is accepted, it has to have the explicit agreement of the purchasers. This is for two reasons. Firstly, they will have to meet any additional cost generated by the scheme in their price for services. Secondly, the regional office of the Management Executive will want to be assured that the capital proposal is consistent with the future plans of the purchasers in terms of the nature and location of services. This check in the system will ensure that inappropriate capital investments are not made.

Having had a business case agreed the trust will receive approval to raise a loan to pay for the project. This loan sanction will be through a mechanism called the external financing limit (EFL). This is an annual limit to the amount of funds the trust can borrow. In essence it represents the gap between the total capital expenditure plan of the trust in the year and the funds it generates internally to contribute to

| **Box 7.6** | |
|---|---|
| **A positive EFL** | The trust needs to borrow money to finance its programme |
| **A negative EFL** | More money is raised by the trust than it needs to finance its programme |
| **Zero EFL** | Capital expenditure is exactly matched by monies generated internally by the trust through its 6% rate of return and changes in working capital balances |

the cost of the programme. It can be a positive or negative figure. Positive implies that loans will be taken. Loans can be obtained from any commercial source, provided it represents best value to the NHS. In practice, loans are arranged through the Treasury as, inevitably, they can obtain the lowest interest rates.

Until 1991 capital was allocated as a one-off grant. There were no loan repayments or interest charges associated with its use. It was, in effect, a free good. In 1991 a system of capital charging was introduced with an aim of making the NHS aware of the cost of the use of capital. It was anticipated that this would lead to a more efficient use of capital. Capital charges are now payable on all capital assets owned and purchased by the NHS. Assets donated through gift or funded from endowments are exempt.

There are two components to capital charges, depreciation and interest. Depreciation is an annual charge that represents the cost of using an asset over its useful life. In the NHS a straight-line basis is used whereby an equal charge is made each year. The NHS uses a predetermined standard useful life for assets. Different types of asset are depreciated over different lengths of time. For example: vehicle, 7 years; computer, 8 years; furniture, 10 years; buildings, up to 80 years. A computer installation costing £240 000 to purchase and with a useful life of 8 years will incur depreciation charges of £30 000 a year. This depreciation charge is a revenue cost and is allowed for in the total cost of the provider. It is as real a cost as payment for drugs or staff.

The second element of capital charges is the interest payments made on loans. Loans are taken at the set-up of a trust to represent the value of the assets transferred from the Secretary of State and for subsequent new expenditure. Each loan will be agreed separately and have an interest rate that represents the then-current market rate. The repayment period of the loan will also be set at the time it is taken, and depend on the circumstances at the time. New loans cannot exceed 20 years. The trust has to repay the principal of the loan in equal parts over its life, and the annual interest. These are revenue costs and are added to the total cost base of the trust.

## CONCLUSION

Financing the NHS is a complex and costly activity at national, regional and local level. While funding overall has increased over and above the rate of inflation for the past 3 years, there can be little doubt that demand for health care has continued to rise also, placing considerable strain on the system and necessitating very skilled financial management.

## REFERENCES

Department of Health (1995) Departmental report, March (Cmd 2812). HMSO, London

NHS Executive (1994) HCHS review: resource allocation 'weighted capitation formula'. HMSO, London

Chartered Institute of Public Finance and Accountancy (1992, 1993, 1994). Health database. CIPFA, London

## FURTHER READING

Perrin J (1988) Resource management in the NHS. Van Nostrand Reinhold in Association with Health Services Management Centre, Wokingham

Ham C (1990) The new National Health Service. Organisation and management. National Association of Health Authorities and Trusts, Radcliffe Medical Press, Oxford

Lilley R (1994) Financial management – a guide for non-financial managers and directors in the NHS. National Association of Health Authorities and Trusts, Radcliffe Medical Press, Oxford

Healthcare Financial Management Association (1995) Introduction to finance in the NHS

Beardsley M, Coles J, Jenkins L (eds) (1987) DRGs and Healthcare. King Edward Hospital Fund for London (1987)

CIPFA/HFMA (1995) Introductory guide to NHS finance in the UK. CIPFA, London

CIMA (1995) NHS funds flow: a guide. CIMA, London

Department of Health (1995) NHS trust finance manual (Cmd 2812). HMSO, London

NHS Executive 1994 HCHS revenue resource allocation weighted capitation formula. HMSO, London

University of York (1994) A formula for distributing NHS revenue. Centre for Health Economics, York

# Human resource management within the NHS

Lynn Copcutt

## INTRODUCTION

The greatest asset of any organisation is its human resources and this is particularly true in the labour-dependent health service. Successful management of the human resource must ensure that employees are selected carefully, that their abilities are used to best effect and that they develop to their full potential. The health service of today requires staff who are highly skilled, adaptable and willing to accept responsibility for the achievement of organisational goals and targets. NHS trusts have to respond quickly to the demands of the market; they therefore have to develop a workforce able to meet this challenge. This chapter deals with those issues that are essential for the development of such a workforce and reviews how the National Health Service is using human resource management to manage and develop its staff.

### Human resource management

Human resource management (HRM) is a strategic approach to management that seeks to maximise the contribution made by the workforce in the achievement of the organisation's goals. Pettigrow & Whipp (1991) offer this further definition: 'Human resource management relates to the total set of knowledge skills and attitudes that firms need to compete. It involves concern for and action in the management of people including selection, training and development, and employee relations.'

Human resource management is more than just another style of management, it is a philosophy that an organisation identifies with. It involves strategic action by management to create a culture that believes employees are valuable assets in which to invest time and money. Such a culture will in turn ensure the commitment of the workforce to the organisation and will promote the release of creativity and innovation. The aims of human resource management can be summarised as follows:

- To create a culture that recognises the contribution made by individuals to the overall achievement of the organisation
- To foster a climate that generates creativity and innovation
- To ensure that individuals maximise their full potential through identifying the needs of the workforce in tandem with strategic and operational planning
- To promote quality through a skilled flexible and committed workforce

## STAFF DEVELOPMENT

'Human resource management is essentially a business orientated philosophy concerning the management of people in order to obtain added value from them and thus achieve a competitive advantage' (Armstrong 1993, p 20).

If management is to achieve added value from staff the organisation must take seriously its staff development function. The implementation of the health service reforms and the introduction of the competitive market within health care has ensured that most organisations are now taking very seriously the development and training activity they provide for their staff. As the business planning process becomes more sophisticated and marketing assumes greater importance it is imperative that staff are equipped with the skills and knowledge to achieve the organisation's objectives. When considering training and development, an organisation needs to take into account how much it is likely to cost, what resources already exist that can be built upon and what priorities need to be satisfied. This means that anyone who is a manager of staff needs to take full responsibility for the learning and development needs of their team members, to ensure that they are being used to their full capacity and that no untapped potential is left unexploited. It also places on managers a key responsibility to keep themselves informed and to contribute towards the development of business objectives so that they can be sure that their staff can deliver the product or service promised.

Once the organisation has decided upon its main priorities and a business plan has been written, the organisation has to ensure that it has a skilled and knowledgeable workforce to deliver its core business. To achieve this a training needs analysis may be conducted.

**Training needs analysis**

A training needs analysis involves collecting data relating to the specific educational and developmental needs of employees. These needs are role-related and should address both the present and future demands of the post-holder. A training needs analysis can be conducted in a variety of ways. The *survey approach* is the most frequently used method of obtaining information. All staff or a representative sample of staff are interviewed or respond by questionnaire to specific questions relating to their role and the development or training they require to conduct that role safely and effectively both now and in the foreseeable future. A training needs analysis could also use the *key informant approach*, which as the name implies collects information concerning the needs of the group from key individuals who are presumed to be in a position to know those needs. These key informants would be representatives of different groups and grades of employee and the focus group technique may be used to collect the relevant data. Finally, information may be obtained from records or reports and in the case of assessing training needs, data may be obtained from individual performance review documentation; this approach is known as the *indicators approach*.

The final stage of any training needs analysis is to make recommendations in the form of a staff development plan or strategy. This often entails prioritising action to ensure that the corporate objectives of the organisation are met within available resources. One could argue that developing and training staff and developing a business plan is a bit like trying to answer the question 'Which came first, the chicken or the egg?'. Does the organisation commit to delivering a product or service before ensuring that its staff have the skills to deliver? Or does the organisation commit itself to developing staff before delivering the service? In reality the answer is usually a little of both. As most health-care organisations move towards the achievement of trust status, there will be an increasing pressure to continue the core business while at the same time developing new areas of service provision in response to market demand. This will ultimately mean that the trust will be relying on the old skills of the staff but will also be looking to develop new ones.

---

**Activity 8.1**

- Review your current role and identify your own development/training needs
- Identify future developments likely to affect your role
- Construct your own personal development plan

---

## The value and purpose of staff development

All individuals have the potential to develop spontaneously and to change over time; it must therefore be the aim of every organisation to harness this capacity and to channel it in the most advantageous direction for both the individual and the organisation. The value of staff development to the organisation encompasses three major factors. Firstly, staff development is an essential part of manpower planning and the realisation of an appropriate skill mix. Manpower planning within an NHS trust must take cognisance of the business plan and the corporate objectives of the trust when identifying its present and future manpower needs. The trust that identifies future manpower needs in conjunction with a progressive staff development programme is the trust that is most likely to respond most competitively within the market place.

Secondly, a comprehensive commitment to staff development is one of the main factors in the maintenance of a contented and stable workforce and serves as a positive aid to recruitment. The secret of using staff development as a means of enhancing morale is to achieve an optimum balance of staff development in line with the opportunities available for job advancement or enrichment within the organisation. Staff should not be prepared for promotions that are never likely to happen; staff not being prepared to meet the challenge of new developments is also counterproductive. The skill of management must be to organise its development programme in line with the opportunities available.

Finally, the commitment of an organisation to staff development will inevitably improve the quality of product or service provided. In the case of an NHS trust this means that by investing in people the quality of patient care will inevitably improve. It is this premise that underpins the Investor in People initiative that has been spearheaded by the Training and Enterprise Councils (TECs). 'Investors in People is based on the experiences of many UK companies which have proved that performance is improved by a planned approach to: setting and communicating business goals and developing people to meet these goals so that what people can do and are motivated to do matches what the business needs them to do' (Investor in People 1991a).

Many NHS trusts are seeking to become an Investor in People organisation. To do this they are assessed against an agreed national standard. The national standard embraces four principles:

- Commitment
- Planning
- Action
- Evaluation

It is called a national standard because it is nationally recognised as the benchmark to which all organisations must work and be successfully assessed before they can be publicly recognised as an Investor in People organisation. The standard is described fully in Box 8.1.

The value of staff development to the individual is enormous and can be identified as follows:

- It promotes a sense of self actualisation and allows the individual to maximise her/his full potential
- It fosters confidence by ensuring competence
- It prepares the individual for future role developments
- It prepares the individual for change and therefore reduces resistance
- It allows the individual to cope with stress more effectively
- It encourages the individual to be involved in her/his own career progression

**Box 8.1** A brief for top managers (Investor in People 1991b)

*National standard for effective investment in people*

An *Investor in People* makes a public commitment from the top to develop all employees to achieve its business objectives.

- Every employer should have a written but flexible plan which sets out business goals and targets, considers how employees will contribute to achieving the plan and specifies how development needs in particular will be assessed and met
- Management should develop and communicate to all employees a vision of where the organisation is going and the contribution employees will make to its success, involving employee representatives as appropriate

An *Investor in People* regularly reviews the training and development needs of all employees.

- The resources for training and developing employees should be clearly identified in the business plan
- Managers should be responsible for regularly agreeing training and development needs with employee in the context of business objectives, setting targets and standards linked, where appropriate, to the achievement of National Vocational Qualifications (or relevant units) and, in Scotland, Scottish Vocational Qualifications

An *Investor in People* takes action to train and develop individuals on recruitment and throughout their employment.

- Action should focus on the training needs of all new recruits and continually developing and improving the skills of existing employees
- All employees should be encouraged to contribute to identifying and meeting their own job-related development needs

An *Investor in People* evaluates the investment in training and development to assess achievement and improve future effectiveness.

- The investment, the competence and commitment of employees, and the use made of skills learned should be reviewed at all levels against business goals and targets
- The effectiveness of training and development should be reviewed at the top level and lead to renewed commitment and target setting

---

**Activity 8.2**

Reflect on your most recent staff development activity. To what extent did it achieve the benefits listed above?

## Approaches to staff development

Health-care organisations have a tendency to view staff development only in the form of the formal courses attended by staff. From the organisation's perspective this makes the development and training activity easy to evaluate. A breakdown is provided at the end of the financial year giving details of the number and type of courses attended and a judgement is then made as to the cost benefit of this investment to the organisation. However formal education is only one way to develop staff. Other ways in which staff may receive development include:

- *Work shadowing:* This is where an individual is given an opportunity to follow another member of staff around in their day-to-day activity to learn what they do, or to give them an appreciation of the effect their work has on someone else, e.g. a health records clerk shadowing a clinic receptionist. The clerk would normally sort the notes out for the clinic, but s/he does not have a true appreciation of what could happen if s/he does not do the job properly unless s/he sees the possible implications for her/himself. Shadowing is also useful when staff are undertaking professional qualifications and may perhaps need to do project work in a different work area.

- *Secondments:* This is where an opportunity is given for a specified time, e.g. 3–6 months, to undertake a specific project, or an opportunity is given for an individual to spend time in a completely different work area, e.g. a secondment for a laboratory officer to work on a marketing project for 3 months. The secondment is usually a very effective means of staff development and at the end of the secondment period the employee returns to her/his own post.

- *Open learning:* Many staff are now taking advantage of the various forms of learning materials now available on the market, through either computer-based training packages, videos or distance learning materials. This flexible approach to learning has two advantages: firstly, the member of staff can choose a topic of their own choice and study in their own time; secondly, the time lost from work is reduced, and this may therefore be more attractive to managers who are having to balance the needs of the organisation with the needs of the individual.

- *Group learning:* This involves all learning that takes place within a group context. The individual needs are identified early in the programme and the programme of activities is organised to meet the needs of the individuals within the group. These techniques are often used to develop interpersonal, group dynamics and team-building skills. They have, however, been more recently used for developing problem-solving skills through the medium of action learning sets.

• *Planned experience:* This is the most common form of staff development within organisations and probably the most effective. Staff undertake a planned period of experience, working usually under the supervision of an experienced member of staff who acts as their mentor or preceptor. The United Kingdom Central Council for Nursing, Midwifery and Health Visiting, in the Post-Registration Education for Practice Project (PREPP – UKCC 1990) identified the need for all nursing, midwifery and health-visiting staff to undergo a period of preceptorship immediately following registration to the profession and when assuming a new role. This proposal was accepted by the Government in 1994 and an implementation date was set for April 1995. For this period of experience to be effective the member of staff should have a clear understanding of the learning outcomes to be achieved from the experience and should receive regular and accurate feedback on her/his performance.

---

**Activity 8.3**

Reconsider the personal development plan you devised for yourself as part of Activity 8.1 in light of the additional information above.
   What changes can you now make that will enhance your development plan?

---

## The external and internal influences on staff development

When assessing the staff development needs of a member of staff consideration should be given to three equally important elements:

• The needs of the organisation
• The needs of the individual
• The needs of the job

The needs of the organisation, the individual and the job will in turn be influenced by both internal and external factors. These factors make a useful check list when planning either your own development

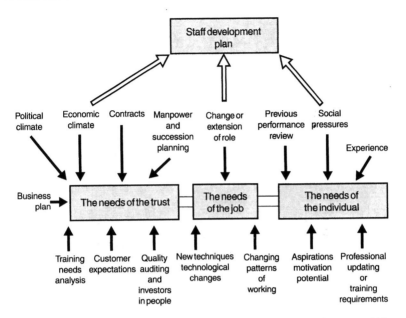

**Fig 8.1** The external and internal factors that influence staff development within an NHS hospital trust

or that of a staff member. A diagrammatic summary is presented in Figure 8.1.

## PERFORMANCE APPRAISAL

Staff development and performance appraisal should be very closely linked. Appraisal has two functions: to recognise in a formal way the contribution an individual member of staff gives to the organisation and to identify development and training needs that will further enhance that contribution. Torrington & Hall (1987, p 403) offer the following definition of Appraisal: 'We all constantly appraise, consciously and unconsciously, objectively and subjectively. When we appraise something we rate its worth, its usefulness and the degree to which it displays various qualities. We appraise ourselves and other people, we appraise behaviour personality and systems. Organisational appraisal systems are an attempt to formalise these activities for the benefit of the individual and the organisation.' It is apparent from this definition that appraisal has two purposes: to benefit the organisation and to benefit the individual (Fig. 8.2).

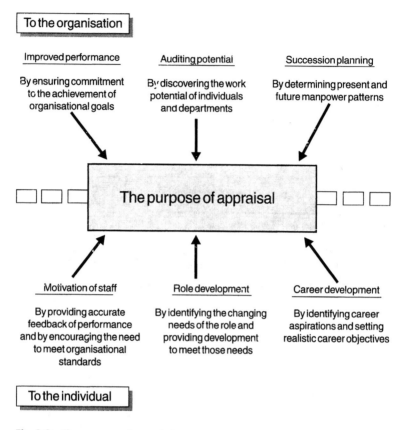

**Fig 8.2** The purpose of appraisal

## The benefits of performance appraisal to the organisation

### Improvement of performance

Effective systems of individual performance review are known to enhance the quality of the product or service provided. Review is the ideal time to encourage team members to commit themselves to objectives that will help towards the achievement of the organisation's overall aims and objectives. Review systems, however, need to address two fundamental issues if they are to have the desired effect of improving performance. Firstly, the objectives should be agreed not imposed; this will ensure a commitment to achieve providing the environment is favourable and the objectives have been carefully constructed. The mnemonic SMART is a useful guide in the formulation of objectives, which should be:

- Specific
- Measurable
- Achievable
- Realistic
- Timebound

Secondly, appraisal should not just review past performance, but should also be seen as an opportunity to look forward and assess the future needs of the individual, ensuring compatibility with the future needs of the organisation.

### Audit of potential

Appraisal offers managers the opportunity to discover the potential that exists within the organisation. Innovation is brought about by individuals who, through using skill, imagination and creativity, generate new and novel ideas in response to market demand. Appraisal allows an audit of this potential to be made and it will draw management's attention to new areas of expertise that should be developed. Managers in these interviews should be looking to identify potential and to allow individual members of staff to become empowered from the lowest levels of the organisation up to and including senior management.

### Succession planning

Appraisal provides an ideal opportunity to assess the potential of staff with respect to the future developments of the organisation. Staff development is costly on both time and money; it would therefore seem sensible that after investing in staff every attempt should be made to retain them within the organisation. Succession planning is about developing your own staff to meet the future human resource needs of the organisation. Succession planning is discussed in more detail later in this chapter.

## The benefits of performance appraisal to the individual

### Increased motivation

Appraisal is about motivating staff to achieve; however it is important to remember that an appraisal that is badly conducted can be a demotivator and prevent the maximisation of potential. Much depends upon the skill of the appraiser in making the process a positive experience for the appraisee. Training is essential to ensure that the appraiser identifies with the system of appraisal used by the organisation and has the necessary skills and knowledge to ensure a fruitful outcome.

## Role development

Appraisal should provide sensitive and accurate feedback to staff about their performance. The appraisee can therefore become a more able performer by identifying her/his strengths and by understanding what changes are needed to further enhance her/his performance. The appraisal interview provides an opportunity to discuss all aspects of the appraisee's role; this is important as roles are constantly changing within the current work climate. These changes bring training and development needs which should be discussed and agreed at appraisal.

## Career development

Performance appraisal provides the opportunity to discuss the career intentions of the appraisee. At appraisal individuals can formulate their career objectives, which if skilfully handled by the appraiser will ensure both confidence and realism – confidence to aim high tempered by the realism that recognises limitations.

## Approaches to staff appraisal
### Management by objectives (MBO)

Management by objectives focuses on actual work performance, it involves goal setting by both employee and manager and it should be a continuous process rather than a one-off event. For this reason MBO should work in conjunction with a dynamic staff development programme.

The limitations of the system are, firstly, that it is very time-consuming, as goal setting requires considerable discussion between appraisee and appraiser, and, secondly, that goal accomplishment is often influenced by factors outside the employee's control, such as resources, finance, performance of colleagues, etc. MBO can provide rather a narrow view of the appraisee's performance because objectives require to be measurable when they are used within the context of appraisal; this implies that there is an emphasis on quantification and less regard is paid to the qualitative aspects of performance. This limitation, however, can be overcome by setting expected standards of achievement or performance indicators for each objective that are dynamic to the appraisee and are qualitative as well as quantitative in nature. This requirement to set levels of performance as targets for achievement is more fully embraced by the behavioural approaches to appraisal.

### Behavioural approaches to appraisal

In an attempt to make appraisal more objective and to reduce appraiser subjectivity and bias, some appraisal schemes have incorporated statements of expected performance. Behavioural expectation scaling (BES) or behaviourally anchored rating scales (BARS) are examples of such an approach. In BES and BARS, the numbers or adjectives of traditional performance rating scales have been replaced by actual descriptions of behaviour. BARS are vertical scales of role specific behaviour. Usually, three to four specific statements or anchors describe sample behaviours for each role dimension. Role dimensions are broad groups of duties or responsibilities. A position or role is broken down into component dimensions and within each specified dimension an ordinal scale is created that reflects job performances from poor to excellent. The appraiser is required to select the statement that best reflects the performance of the appraisee for that dimension of the role. (See Box 8.2 for an example of how the Midwifery Department of an NHS trust has utilised behavioural scales within their appraisal documentation.)

Behaviour approaches to appraisal are very time consuming to develop, as they are role-specific and therefore require to be individually designed. They are also dynamic documents in that they require to be updated as role changes occur. They do, however, seem to be well accepted both by appraiser and appraisee, who welcome the security of knowing the expected level of performance to be achieved.

Whatever type of performance review system is used, it is imperative that it is introduced sensitively into the organisation with the full cooperation of the staff. Providing this is achieved the results will be positive. Evidence from the motivation theorists, Hertzberg et al (1959) and Mayo (1975), suggests that money will get people to work but does not necessarily mean they will stay. A feeling of being valued and useful is much more important if the organisation is to achieve long-term commitment from its staff.

**Box 8.2**  A behavioural approach to appraisal

The Midwifery Department of the City Hospital NHS Trust in Birmingham have incorporated a simple behavioural scale into their appraisal documentation. The role of the E Grade midwife has been broken down into four dimensions. Each of these main dimensions was further broken down into subdimensions and behavioural scales were written for each subdimension. The example offered below represents two subdimensions within the management section.

| Management skills | Self | Manager | Comments |
|---|---|---|---|
| **Ward/Unit organisation**<br>Calmly and efficiently manages the ward/unit in the absence of the midwife/nurse-in-charge. | | | |
| Organisational skills are developing well.<br>Lacks motivation to develop organisational skills. | | | |
| Unable to organise the ward/unit efficiently. | | | |
| **Communication**<br>Communicates effectively with all levels of staff. | | | |
| Generally communicates effectively. Sometimes lacks awareness of the need to communicate. | | | |
| Attitude sometimes prevents good communication. | | | |
| Fails to recognise the importance of communication, therefore poor communication. | | | |

## Manpower planning

Most, if not all writings on manpower planning attempt to define the meaning of the term; this inevitably leads to an open-ended debate which is never fully resolved. What is important, however, is the 'planning' element. Manpower planning is a strategic matter in the sense that there is a determination of objectives and an intent to meet them. An over-riding factor in manpower planning within the current NHS is the need to provide high-quality, cost-effective care.

Manpower planning is the approach to the management of human resources based on an anticipation of the future needs of an organisation and the behavioural patterns of individuals within it. The actual practice of manpower planning can be viewed as the balancing of the demand for labour with the supply. This balancing can involve a number of policies and techniques – recruitment, training, return to work and deployment are examples. The manpower planning process can be divided into three main components (Fig. 8.3):

- Determining the *demand* for staff
- Assessing how these staff will be *supplied*
- Deciding how a *balance* between demand and supply can be modelled

There is often some confusion between manpower planning and skill mix and it is important to emphasise that the two are not the same. Skill mix is a technique to be used within the demand side of the equation. One means of determining the demand for staff is to undertake a skill mix review to assess what categories of staff are required and what qualifications they should possess to work in a particular area. This process, however, does not deal with the practicalities of how you would, or indeed whether it is possible to, supply the staff to meet this demand; this is the remit of the manpower planners. The issue of skill mix will be explored in greater depth later in this chapter.

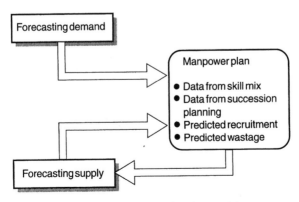

**Fig 8.3**  A manpower planning model

If skill mix is a technique on the demand side of our equation then 'succession planning' can be viewed as a technique on the supply side. One means of ensuring that an organisation's future requirements for particular skills, knowledge and competencies are met is to successfully manage the careers of its existing staff. How to manage the careers of their staff, however, is an issue that many employers struggle to come to terms with.

The following sections will attempt to explore in more detail how both skill mix and succession planning can be effectively used within the manpower planning process.

## Manpower planning activities

At this point it is worth exploring the manpower planning activities carried out at various levels within an NHS trust. At ward level a manager is concerned to ensure that the duty rotas allow for 24-hour cover and that any on-call arrangements are not compromised by sickness, absence, maternity leave, annual leave or study leave. At directorate level there will be a shift of emphasis on to the longer term, with attention being given to reducing staff overlaps and the need to recruit staff that can meet the changing demands of the directorate as it responds to contractual requirements and consumer demand. At trust Board level, manpower concerns will be strategic in nature and will encompass such issues as training and education, the requirements of professional bodies and training commissions and the need to ensure that business plans and manpower plans are developed in coordination with each other.

## Skill mix

Skill mix has been defined by Nerssling (1990) as:

> the balance between trained and untrained, qualified and unqualified and supervisory and operative staff within a service area as well as between different staff groups. . . . optimum skill mix is achieved when the desired standard of service is provided at the minimum cost, which is consistent with the efficient deployment of trained, qualified and supervisory personnel and the maximisation of contributions from all staff members. It will ensure the best possible use of scarce professional skills to maximise the service to clients.

From this definition there are a number of key points to be made.

- Skill mix includes the identification of the different range of tasks and responsibilities required

- Potential staffing needs should not be defined in terms of current grading systems
- It looks at the potential 'mix' of professional staff required; this means challenging the boundaries of where one staff group meets another
- Finally, by challenging current grade definitions and the boundaries that exist between staff groups, the process becomes zero-based; in other words, when entering into skill mix reviews one should have no preconceived ideas of grades and groups required

At this point it is worth reiterating the difference between skill mix and grade mix. Skill mix crosses staff groups while grade mix looks at grades within a particular group. The process of assessing skill mix can be broken down into several stages:

1. Define the client group
2. Define the type of health care required by this group
3. Define the responsibilities and the general blend of skills required
4. Define what type of staff and how many of each group are required
5. Determine the appropriate job descriptions, training systems, and recruitment and selection procedures

All of these stages, except the last one, are wholly concerned with specifying or determining demand for staff. They involve planning the organisation's future staff requirements; they do not, however, apart from the last stage, concern themselves with how the staff may be supplied in order to satisfy that demand. In manpower planning terms only one side of the demand/supply equation has been determined. It is only when supply is in equilibrium with demand that the desired balance will be achieved.

It would be wrong to see skill mix and manpower planning as a one-off exercise. Manpower planning, as with business planning, or indeed any type of planning, is an ongoing process. There is no ultimate end, merely a continuous balancing of demand and supply. This is very apparent to those who strive to balance the 24-hour needs of an NHS trust hospital with the numbers of professionally qualified staff available to the NHS.

Not only is skill mix an ongoing process, it is also a reflective activity. It continually forces us to challenge long-held convictions about the way jobs are constructed and how health care is provided. By being innovative in determining the skill mix required we ensure the best possible use of scarce professional skills to maximise the service to clients.

## Succession planning

There are close parallels between management development and succession planning. Both activities imply that a conscious attention is given by the organisation to the issue of career development. Both techniques seek to ensure that vacancies in the future are filled by the employees of today; succession planning, however, is seen as a far more prescriptive way of tracking and elevating staff through a clear career hierarchy. In this age of leaner and flatter organisations with an emphasis on horizontal rather than vertical relationships and with jobs changes demanding different skills, management development techniques may replace or run parallel to succession planning.

The management of 'careers' is an extremely difficult part of manpower planning. Career opportunity development in itself is not an independent part of an organisation's activity: to a greater or lesser extent the career opportunities of staff will be determined by the organisation's future manpower requirements, i.e. its demand for staff. This point is clearly demonstrated when an organisation moves towards a more flexible and fluid workforce. When jobs and roles are classified in terms of core (permanent) and non-core (temporary or fixed-term) career development opportunities can either be dashed completely or moved to the periphery along with job security. This reclassification of jobs forces individuals to think in terms of skills retraining and holding a 'portfolio' of jobs, as opposed to having one full-time post and a career. This must prompt organisations to reconsider their whole approach to succession planning. Long-term succession planning is possible in stable or slowly changing organisations. When looking at jobs it is possible to highlight possible future successors and to identify the career development opportunities required to do those jobs. However one should always question whether the job will exist in the future and if it does whether the job requirements and selection criteria will be the same.

In summary, it can be argued that manpower planning is a continuous exercise that is concerned with meeting the demands of an organisation for a supply of staff. It involves, firstly, assessing demand for staff, and this may be achieved through the determination of skill mix. It is essential that skill mix is approached from a zero-based perspective to ensure that the staff profile that results is matched to the organisation's objectives and not merely an altered image of what has gone before. Determination of demand is only one side of the equation and must lead to determining how that demand will be met, i.e. supplied. Succession planning is one way of achieving this aim, as it seeks to manage the career pathways of employees to ensure that the future manpower needs of the organisation are met largely from the existing workforce.

---

**Activity 8.4**

Select a small section of the organisation to which you belong, e.g. ward or department.

- List the total activities of the section
- Using a zero base (i.e. without reference to current staffing) identify the professional and ancillary staff needed to fulfil those activities

---

## EQUAL OPPORTUNITIES IN EMPLOYMENT

The United Kingdom is a multiracial society in which women account for nearly half of the working population and increasingly those with disabilities are being recognised as able to make a full contribution to working life. However, it is often people from these groups who experience unfair and unlawful discrimination in employment. This is not only unlawful, but it is also bad for the organisation. In order to be successful in today's competitive environment, employers need to actively encourage, recruit and develop the best available employees regardless of race, sex or disability.

### Relevant legislation

Equal opportunities is a natural and integral part of good management practice which is aimed at developing employees to the fullest extent possible for the benefit of the organisation and themselves. Various pieces of legislation exist to provide people with some protection from unfair discrimination and to make employers aware of their legal responsibilities. These are summarised as follows:

**The Sex Discrimination Act 1975 and 1986** states that it is unlawful to discriminate directly or indirectly on the grounds of sex or marital status, or to apply requirements or conditions that have a disproportionately advantageous effect on people of a particular sex or marital status where these cannot be justified. It also states that it is unlawful to apply pressure to discriminate or to aid discrimination by another person. Exceptions to this could apply in some positions, where there are genuine occupational requirements and an employer may stipulate the sex or race.

**The Race Relations Act 1976** states that it is unlawful to discriminate directly or indirectly on the grounds of race or ethnic origin, or to apply requirements or conditions which have a disproportionately advantageous effect on people of a particular race or ethnic origin where these cannot be justified. It also states that it is unlawful to apply pressure to discriminate or to aid discrimination by another person.

**The Equal Pay Act 1970** states that it is unlawful to treat an employee of one sex less favourably in respect of pay or terms and conditions of employment than an employee of the opposite sex who does the same or broadly similar work.

**The Disabled Persons (Employment) Acts 1944 and 1958** provide specific provision for the employment of people with disabilities. The quota scheme states that employers with more than 20 employees should employ 3% of registered disabled people in their workforce. In practice this legislation is poorly upheld and it is by encouragement rather than enforcement that it is applied. However, Parliament is currently considering a new bill similar in provision to the Sex Discrimination and Race Relations Acts.

**The Rehabilitation of Offenders Act 1974** (exemption orders 1975 and 1986) states that if no further offences are committed and considering the severity of the sentence imposed, a person has a right to class her/his conviction as spent following a stated period of time. This means that s/he does not have to declare it on application forms. 'Spent' sentences should not be used to exclude people from employment or promotion. However, in certain occupations, such as nursing, any convictions regardless of time and severity have to be disclosed.

## Types of discrimination

People may feel discriminated against for many reasons. These reasons usually include sex, race, colour, nationality, ethnic origin, disability, marital status, sexual orientation, responsibility for dependants, trade union or political activities, religious beliefs and being HIV-positive or suffering from AIDS. There are several types of discrimination and they are defined as follows.

**Direct discrimination** is when one person is treated less favourably than another person for any of the above reasons, e.g. it is unlawful to refuse a woman employment in a job traditionally held by a man.

**Indirect discrimination** occurs when a requirement or condition that cannot be justified is applied equally to everyone, but has the effect in practice of disadvantaging a considerably higher proportion of one group of people than another. The inability to comply would have a detrimental effect such as not being selected for a post or offered promotion, e.g. an upper age limit of 28 for a post can be indirectly discriminatory to women as many women have career breaks to bring up children.

**Victimisation** occurs when a person is given less favourable treatment, when, for example they have brought proceedings or given evidence in a case of discrimination. This only applies where information was given in good faith; false allegations will render the victimisation claim invalid.

**Harassment** is any behaviour, deliberate or otherwise, directed at an individual that is offensive, threatening or intimidating.

### Developing an equal opportunities policy

One of the first essential steps in ensuring an equal opportunities culture is to develop a policy that includes guidelines for good practice in respect of recruitment and selection, career development and training, grievance and discipline. A policy is not an end in itself but it does provide a framework for action and monitoring. Box 8.3 gives an example of an equal opportunities policy statement within the NHS.

In order for the equal opportunities policy to be successful it should outline the responsibilities of both managers and employees toward equal opportunities. Monitoring of the policy to ensure effective

**Box 8.3** Equal opportunities in employment: policy statement

The Royal Wolverhampton Hospitals NHS trust recognises that all forms of discrimination are unacceptable. This policy has been introduced to provide equality of opportunity in employment for all job applicants and employees by eliminating all discrimination – direct and indirect – victimisation and harassment.

By enforcing this policy the aim is to ensure no job applicant or employee receives less favourable treatment on grounds of sex, race, colour, nationality, ethnic or national origin, disability, marital status, sexual orientation, responsibility for dependants, age, trade union or political activities, religious beliefs, being HIV Positive or having AIDS, or is disadvantaged by any conditions or requirements which cannot be justified.

All areas of employment are affected – recruitment and selection, training and career development, grievance and disciplinary procedures, and terms and conditions of service.

The Trust aims to make full use of the talents and resources of all employees and to establish a culture which promotes a good and productive working environment. The commitment to providing the best for the people who use the Trust can only be achieved if the workforce is reflective of the population of the area served.

Procedures arising from this policy will continually be monitored to assess their effectiveness. Any defects will be corrected immediately and the policy amended and improved as required.

It is the responsibility of all staff to be aware of the contents of this policy and work to them at all times.

The Royal Wolverhampton Hospitals NHS Trust – working with you to promote equality of opportunity.

implementation is essential. The monitoring process should involve the collection and classification of information regarding the ethnic origin, gender, etc of all current employees and potential employees applying for a job. It is only by monitoring and analysing the data that evidence of discrimination can be detected. The data may reveal that individuals from specific groups are not recruited, fail to achieve promotion, or are recruited in significantly lower numbers than the level of applications would suggest. It may also be evident that some groups are under-represented in some departments or on some shifts. When such evidence is apparent within an organisation it must be the role of management to investigate the possible causes and take steps to ensure it is rectified.

## RECRUITMENT AND SELECTION

The majority of managers are frequently involved in the recruitment and selection of potential employees. In line with equal opportunities legislation, the aim of management should be to recruit in a fair and systematic manner in order to get the right person for the job. Mistakes can be extremely costly both to the organisation and to the individual. It is expensive both in the financial cost incurred and also in the effort and stress it can put on all concerned. Ideally all managers should undergo training in recruitment and selection techniques and should ensure that all applicants throughout the process are assessed against job-related criteria that can be justified. Each applicant should be assessed according to her/his capability to carry out the job. No general assumptions or prejudgements should be made by managers regarding the suitability of a person for a particular job or whether they will 'fit in'. An unbiased approach should always be adopted and a job must never be thought of as 'man's work' or 'women's work'.

### The recruitment and selection process

The recruitment and selection process is summarised in Box 8.4. Different aspects of that process, however, require more detailed discussion and explanation.

### The job description

The first essential step to recruitment and selection is to draw up a job description that clearly defines the job purpose and highlights the key duties and responsibilities. A job description should include:

- The job title
- The location and department in which the post is based
- The lines of accountability
- A job summary
- A description of the main duties and responsibilities

### Person specification criteria

Person specification criteria are used within the recruitment and selection process to ensure fairness and to reduce interviewer bias and subjectivity at both the shortlisting and formal interview stage. To that end they must be agreed and used by all involved in the selection process and made clear to potential candidates. In formulating the

**Box 8.4** The recruitment and selection process

Identify job vacancy
↓
Review job description
↓
Reassess job in line with organisational needs
↓
Rewrite the job description
↓
Determine person specification
↓
Draft advertisement
↓
Advertise internally and externally
↓
Shortlist candidates
↓
Conduct formal interview
↓
Check references and health assessment of candidates
↓
Inform candidates of outcome
↓
Offer post–interview counselling to unsuccessful candidates
↓
Plan induction programme for successful candidate

criteria, reference must be made to the job description, which serves as a guide in the determination of the knowledge, skills and abilities needed to fulfil the post. The criteria usually fall into two categories: those that are essential for the post and those that are desirable or advantageous (see Box 8.5 for an example proforma). When constructing the person specification criteria it is important that all the statements are clear and nothing is left to the interpretation of the reader. All the criteria should be written in such a way that they are measurable and can be weighted to indicate their importance to the successful fulfilment of the role. The job description and the person specification are the crucial elements in the selection and interviewing process; it is important that they are carefully constructed and that they are a true account of the requirements of the post. In this age of extreme competition within the arena of work, managers can be called to justify their selection decisions; it should not be at this point that anomalies are discovered.

---

**Activity 8.5**

Using the sample proforma in Box 8.5, devise the person specification criteria for your current post.

---

### Recruitment advertising

The job description and person specification must be used to underpin the recruitment advertisement as this ensures continuity in the selection process. Careful attention must also be paid to the accuracy of information and the setting of an appropriate time scale, e.g. the placing of the advert and the dates for shortlisting and interview must be coordinated carefully. Consideration must be given to the publication or journal used to advertise the position to ensure maximum attention from suitable candidates. The advert must indicate a point of contact within the organisation from whom information relating to the post may be easily obtained. Recruitment agencies and professional organisations and societies can be a valuable source of advice in the recruitment of suitably qualified staff.

### The shortlisting process

Following the closing date the applications received should be considered against the person specification criteria drawn up for the post. Staff who will be involved in the interviewing stage should be involved in the shortlisting process. The reason for rejecting any applicants should be stated clearly and records of this decision on a

**Box 8.5** Personal specification proforma

| Attributes | Essential | Advantageous |
|---|---|---|
| Education/qualifications | | |
| Professional qualifications | | |
| Experience | | |
| Job-related skills/aptitudes | | |
| Interpersonal skills | | |
| Other requirements | | |

shortlisting report form. Sometimes there may be an above-average number of applications meeting the criteria for the post; in this instance managers may consider using other selection methods which act as the preliminary assessment and reduce the number of applicants that will proceed to the formal interview. Such alternative methods may include a preliminary interview, a presentation on a relevant topic or a report or paper on a related subject. Whatever method is used it should be fair, consistent and assessed against the person specification criteria.

### The formal interview

**Before the interview** it is important to ensure adequate time is provided for it. An appropriate venue should be arranged that allows for minimum interruption and the date should be agreed with the key players in the interview. A minimum of two persons should always be involved. All the information likely to be required by the candidates should be determined and made available. A pleasant waiting area should also be identified for the candidates.

**During the interview** candidates should be asked appropriate questions designed to test the person specification criteria and the relevant responses and comments should be recorded on an assessment form. All candidates should be allowed the opportunity to ask questions of the panel and informed of the arrangements for telling them of the outcome of the panel's decision.

**After the interview** all the notes should be clearly recorded and the views of all the interviewers sought to ensure a fair decision. The successful candidate should be told as soon as possible and the unsuccessful candidates should be informed and offered post-interview counselling. It is imperative that all records of the interview are retained by the organisation for a minimum of 12 months. The relevant documentation and contract of employment should then be issued to the successful candidate and an induction programme should be organised.

## CONCLUSION

Organisations become successful organisations when they recognise the value of their workforce. This is particularly so in the National

Health Service where so much depends upon the skill and commitment of its staff. The human resource management philosophy advocates that valuing staff is more than just treating them nicely, it is about creating an organisational culture that embraces the importance of the individual and the need to invest time and money in her/his development. Organisations that are investing in their workforce recognise the need for a staff development programme that is closely linked to performance review and reflects the corporate objectives outlined in the business plan. The human resource of the contemporary health service is a very costly commodity, so it is essential that attention is paid to the careful recruitment and selection of staff and that once employed by the organisation staff must make most use of their skills and expertise. Over recent years manpower planning has become a crucial part of NHS planning at every level. Careful attention must be given to ensure that the correct mix of staff delivers quality care in the most cost-effective way.

## REFERENCES

Armstrong M (1993) Human resource management, strategy and action. Kogan Page, London
Disabled Persons (Employment) Act 1944. HMSO, London
Disabled Persons (Employment) Act 1958. HMSO, London
Equal Pay Act 1970. HMSO, London
Hertzberg F, Mauser B, Snyderman DB (1959) The motivation to work. John Wiley, New York
Investor in People (1991a) The toolkit. Employment Department, Sheffield
Investor in People (1991b) A brief for top managers. Employment Department, Sheffield
Lilley R, Wilson L (1994) The human resources agenda. An action checklist. NAHAT, Radcliffe Medical Press, Oxford
Mayo E (1975) The social problems of industrial civilisation. Routledge & Kegan Paul, London
Pettigrow A, Whipp R (1991) Managing change for competitive success. Blackwell, Oxford
Nerssling R (1990) In: Harrison R 1988 Training and development. IPM, London
Race Relations Act 1976. HMSO, London
Sex Discrimination Act 1975. HMSO, London
Sex Discrimination Act 1986. HMSO, London
Rehabilitation of Offenders Act 1974. HMSO, London
Torrington D, Hall L (1987) Personnel management – a new approach. Prentice Hall, London
UKCC (1990) Post registration education for practice report. United Kingdom Central Council for Nursing, Midwifery and Health Visiting, London

# Quality and standards

*Frances Cooper*

## INTRODUCTION AND BACKGROUND

The maintenance of high standards of care is not a new idea to professionals within the National Health Service; they have always been concerned about the service they provide to patients or clients and have through the years been the principal guardians of service quality. The desire to provide the best possible service to patients was fundamental to the establishment of the professions in the United Kingdom. The professions developed a self-controlling mechanism through the establishment of professional bodies, e.g. the British Medical Association, the General Nursing Council, the Central Midwives Board. These bodies influenced quality through their training, licensing and disciplinary functions and, despite considerable changes to their structure and powers, still do so today. Despite this obvious desire to maintain a good service the issue of quality in the NHS remained implicit rather than explicit until the health-care reforms of the 1980s and early 1990s brought a change of emphasis.

During the 1980s industry in the UK was experiencing an attitudinal change that focused heavily on the need to produce goods and services that would compete favourably in the overseas market. Ideas for improving quality were greatly influenced by the American and Japanese experience of creating a culture of organisational excellence and it was this concept that prompted the Government to launch a

National Quality Campaign in 1984. This campaign established an awareness within both public and private organisations of the need to monitor and control the quality of products and services and to develop systems to do this. The NHS was strongly encouraged by the Government to ensure a quality control system, but initially the ideas met with resistance and scepticism from the professionals, who believed that quality was implicit in the service they provided and that the requirements of industry should not always be applied to the health service. From this initial resistance, a worthy lesson can be learnt about quality and its relevance to the health service: 'Concern about quality of care must be as old as medicine itself, but an honest concern for quality however genuine is not the same as methodical assessment based on reliable evidence' (Maxwell 1985, p 99).

High-quality care is undoubtedly the major aim of the health service, but there is also the need to monitor and prove that aim has been achieved. This has become even more imperative with the advent of the quasi-market in health care and the contracting process between purchasers and providers. Contracts for health care must now stipulate the levels of quality that are expected by the purchasers; this therefore necessitates a comprehensive quality assurance strategy within all provider units. Likewise, the Patient's Charter implemented by the Government in 1991 clearly identifies the rights and standards of service every patient can expect from the health service. This initiative has added consumer pressure to the implementation of quality assurance in the NHS. This chapter will attempt to examine the major issues involved in ensuring a quality service as it applies to an NHS trust; meeting the needs of contracts and the Patient's Charter are two such issues.

### Definitions

Collins Dictionary describes quality as: 'a degree or standard of achievement'. The British Standards Institute defines quality as: 'the totality of feature and characteristics of a product or service that bears on its ability to satisfy stated or applied needs' (British Standards, BS5750). Quality in health services can be defined as: 'fully meeting requirements of lowest cost or more specifically fully meeting the needs of those who need the service most at the lowest cost to the organisation within the limits and directives set by higher authorities and purchasers' (Ovretveit 1992).

---

**Activity 9.1**

Describe in a few words what you understand to be the meaning of 'quality'.

---

The term 'quality' is used in many situations and it often means different things to different people. The following definitions are provided in an attempt to differentiate and clarify the different quality terms used in the NHS.

**Quality assurance**: 'Taking positive action to assess and evaluate performance against agreed and defined standards in order to create and manage a service which regularly achieves desired levels of care or service' (Ball 1989).

**Quality improvement**: 'Quality improvement refers to enhancing the quality of a particular aspect of the service such as improving the quality of access by reducing waiting lists' (Hill et al 1990).

**Quality control**: 'Quality control refers to a methodology for ensuring that specific standards of care are attained' (Five Regional Consortium 1991).

## Total quality management (TQM)

Total quality management acknowledges that all staff within the organisation are fundamental to improving the quality of service provision. It embraces the concept of the quality chain, in that the actions of one member of staff automatically affect one or more members of staff. This chain effect is demonstrated in the case study in Box 9.1.

---

**Box 9.1**  Case study

The Supplies Department of an NHS trust purchases electronic thermometers. The thermometers are supplied to the ward staff, who in themselves are customers of the Supplies Department. The ward staff use the thermometers to monitor and record a patient's temperature – the quality of the thermometer purchased will influence the accuracy of the recording. The accuracy of the recording will influence patient recovery and ultimately patient satisfaction. Thus a quality chain effect is seen to take place.

Total quality management is about getting it right first time by ensuring quality at every level within the organisation. This notion is encompassed within the following definition of TQM: 'A cost effective system for integrating the continuous improvement efforts of people at all levels within an organisation to deliver products and services which ensure customer satisfaction' (Collard et al 1990).

The main elements of TQM are described by Morgan & Everett (1994), using the work of Joiner & Scholtes (1985), and involve three key areas:

- The customer, whose needs are paramount to the determination of quality
- Team work as a means of achieving quality
- A scientific approach to decision-making based on data collection and analysis

Joiner & Scholtes (1985) incorporated these elements into a triangle which has become known as the Joiner Triangle (Fig. 9.1). The customer focus is seen to be centred at the apex of the triangle, signifying the overriding importance of providing a customer-focused service. The following part of this chapter will attempt to relate these elements to the maintenance of quality in the NHS.

## TOTAL QUALITY MANAGEMENT WITHIN THE NHS: CUSTOMER FOCUS

'Patients must always come first' was the message at the heart of the Patient's Charter launched by the Government in (1991) and updated in 1995. This charter, which puts the Citizen's Charter into practice within the NHS, is a practical representation of the Government's drive towards consumerism and a client-led National Health Service. The charter sets out the rights and standards that every patient can expect to receive from the NHS. The charter differentiates between patient rights and expectations in the following way:

- *Rights*: These are standards of service which the patient *will receive all the time*
- *Expectations*: These are standards of service which the NHS *is aiming to achieve*. Exceptional circumstances may prevent these standards being met (Patient's Charter 1991, p 4)

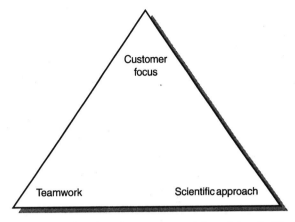

**Fig 9.1** The elements of total quality management (from Joiner & Scholtes 1985)

The charter identifies standards for all sections of the health service, including:

- General practitioner services
- Hospital services
- Community services
- Ambulance services
- Dental, optical and pharmaceutical services
- Maternity services

The overall patient's rights and standards that the NHS is expected to achieve are summarised in Box 9.2.

---

**Box 9.2** Rights and standards throughout the NHS

***Access to services***
Every patient has the *right* to:

- receive health care on the basis of their clinical need, not on their ability to pay, their lifestyle or any other factor
- be registered with a GP and be able to change their GP easily and quickly if they want to
- get emergency medical treatment at any time through their GP, the emergency ambulance service and hospital accident and emergency departments
- be referred to a consultant acceptable to them, when their GP thinks it is necessary, and to be referred for a second opinion if patient and GP agree this is desirable

Every patient can *expect* the NHS to make it easy for everyone to use its services, including children, elderly people or people with physical or mental disabilities.

If a child needs to be admitted to hospital, parents can *expect* them to be cared for in a children's ward under the supervision of a consultant paediatrician. Exceptionally, when a child has to be admitted to a ward other than a children's ward, parents can *expect* a named consultant paediatrician to be responsible for advising on their care.

### Personal consideration and respect

Patients have the *right* to choose whether or not they want to take part in medical research or medical student training.

Patients can *expect* all the staff they meet face to face to wear name badges.

Patients can *expect* the NHS to respect their privacy, dignity and religious and cultural beliefs at all times and in all places. For example, meals should suit their dietary and religious needs. Staff should ask them whether they want to be called by their first or last name and respect their preference.

### Providing information

Patients have the *right* to:

- have any proposed treatment, including any risks involved in that treatment and any alternatives, clearly explained to them before they decide whether to agree to it
- have access to their health records, and to know that everyone working for the NHS is under a legal duty to keep their records confidential
- have any complaint about NHS services (whoever provides them) investigated and to get a quick, full written reply from the relevant chief executive or general manager
- receive detailed information on local health services. This includes information on the standards of service they can expect, waiting times and on local GP services

The rights and expectations identified by the Patient's Charter will be a very important focus of any NHS trust's quality assurance strategy; however, other considerations will include those standards identified in the contracts negotiated with GP fundholders and joint purchasing health authorities (DHAs and FHSAs) (see Table 9.1 for an example).

At this point it becomes evident that there are different perspectives on the word 'customer' as it is applied to the health service. 'The customer' may refer to the patient or the recipient of care, but it can

**Table 9.1** Quality specification for contract year 1995/6: **Directorate/Department** – Professional nursing; **Category** – Nursing practice (Source: Quality Specification for Contracts, Royal Wolverhampton NHS Trust, Wolverhampton)

| Issue/topic | Standard(S)/target(T) | S/T | Monitoring method | Resources |
|---|---|---|---|---|
| An individualised approach will be used to provide nursing care | A first level registered nurse has overall responsibility for the nursing care of each patient | S | Observation of duty rotas and nursing care plans | |
| | All nursing care is documented and signed/countersigned by a Registered Nurse | S | Observation of nursing records using audit and checks by Ward Manager | |
| | All newly admitted patients will have an initial nursing assessment undertaken by a Registered Nurse within 24 hours | S | Observation of nursing records using audit and checks by Ward Manager | |
| | A plan of care, based on the documented initial assessment, will be formulated within 24 hours | S | Observation of nursing records using audit and checks by Ward Manager | |
| | Nursing care plans will be developed from admission to discharge, reflecting ongoing assessment and evaluation | S | Discharge of patients audit and observation of nursing records | |
| | Documented 'goals of care' are measurable and achievable | S | Observation of nursing records | |
| | Care plans are developed in conjunction with the patient and/or informal carer to incorporate their views and wishes | S | Patient/relative interviews/questionnaire | |
| | Registered nurses will monitor the nursing care given in accordance with locally agreed practices and policies | S | Nursing audit | |
| | Nursing staff maintain the patient's rights for courtesy, privacy, dignity and confidentiality at all times | S | Observation<br>Patient interview/questionnaire | |
| | The use of single sex bays within wards will be maintained in line with the Royal College of Nursing guidelines | S | Observation<br>Patient interview | |
| | Ongoing written evaluation reports of patient progress towards achievements of 'goals' are maintained | S | Observation of nursing records | |

also mean the general practitioner or health authority that pays the bill. Meeting customer needs within the health service has been likened to selling shoes to teenagers. The shoe industry has to produce a product that is attractive to the adolescent in that it conforms to fashion trends and yet at the same time takes cognisance of the financial constraints of parents who ultimately pay the bill. NHS trusts therefore require to have a two-pronged approach to quality assurance, addressing the needs of both their patients and their purchasers.

It is important at this point to examine how the needs of the patients or clients may be determined. An NHS trust may seek to determine customer opinion in a variety of ways (Figs 9.2 and 9.3).

## Trust-wide surveys

This will involve consulting the views of patients across the trust. The overall aims of the survey would be twofold:

- To assess the degree of importance that patients place on the different aspects of care they receive
- To assess the degree of satisfaction that patients feel towards the actual care they have received

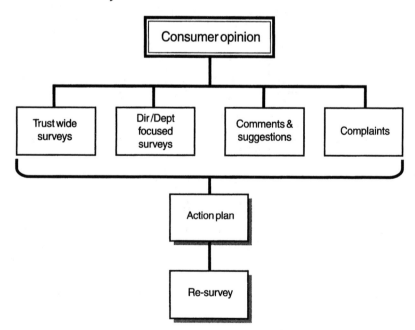

**Fig 9.2** Different ways of determining consumer views within an NHS hospital trust (Royal Wolverhampton NHS Trust, New Cross Hospital, Wolverhampton)

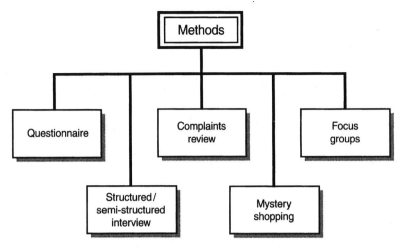

**Fig 9.3** Methods of data collection used by an NHS hospital trust to determine consumer views (Royal Wolverhampton NHS Trust, New Cross Hospital, Wolverhampton)

The survey would involve the use of a questionnaire or structured interviews and is likely to address the general aspects of care that would be pertinent to all wards and departments across the Trust. Consumer views towards the services they receive may also be obtained by a process known as Mystery Shopping; this involves asking someone who is in receipt of health care specifically to observe and report back on specific aspects of service delivery. This observation is often undertaken without health carers' knowledge. Alternatively, a senior person within the organisation (often an executive or non-executive Board member) assumes the role of a relative or patient to monitor aspects of service provision.

## Directorate or departmental focused surveys

This would involve consulting the views of patients within a particular department or directorate. The aims of the survey would be the same as those identified for the trust-wide survey, but specific and relevant to the department or directorate. Questionnaires or structured interviews may be used, but more commonly the focus group technique is utilised. Focus groups are a very effective method of identifying consumer views. A small representative group of patients are assembled to answer questions on a specific topic; in this instance their views regarding the type of service they would wish to see within a department or directorate would be discussed. A facilitator leads the session to ensure that everyone is involved in the discussion.

## Suggestions and comments

The use of suggestion boxes throughout the trust gives both patients and staff the opportunity to offer suggestions for the improvement of care. This method is only successful if patients are made aware of the opportunity to put forward suggestions and are positively encouraged to do so.

## Complaints

The Patient's Charter (1991) informs patients of their right to complain if they are dissatisfied with the care they are receiving or have received. The charter stipulates that the complaint must be acknowledged within two working days and must be dealt with within 1 month in the case of informal complaints and within 6 months for formal complaints. Patients must be made aware of the procedure for making a complaint and assisted to do. All complaints are dealt with and responded to on an individual basis, but an overall review of all complaints is regularly conducted by an NHS trust to determine trends or patterns of dissatisfaction and to suggest the appropriate action that should be taken.

The NHS Executive (EL (95) 121) has recently issued guidance to trusts on the management of complaints. Trusts are required to implement a complaints policy, in line with the guidance, by April 1996.

## Team work

TQM is about the creation of a culture where everyone is aware of the need to continuously examine their work with the view to improving quality for the customer. This individual emphasis on quality performance has a ripple effect along the quality chain that ultimately ensures that a quality service is delivered. This culture of team work has to be created by management: it does not occur naturally. Management firstly need to ensure that the impetus for quality is seen to come from the top and diffuses throughout the organisation. Strategic planning for an NHS trust should reflect the type of quality service the trust would wish to achieve. A quality strategy once it has been agreed should influence operational plans, ensuring individual departments and directorates implement those elements that are appropriate to them. A quality strategy for an NHS trust usually incorporates a quality

---

**Box 9.3** Quality strategy (Source: Royal Wolverhampton NHS Trust)

*Quality statement*
A recognised quality service will 'at all times meet and when possible exceed patients and customer expectation'. In so doing it will clearly demonstrate a commitment to continuous improvement. This commitment will turn what to date have been viewed as failures and problems into opportunities.

Recognising that quality of service will be the deciding factor in the success of the Trust, it is necessary to ensure that those elements that contribute to the quality of service provision are sensibly managed. Quality development has no finite end but should be seen as a journey of continuous improvement. The implemented strategy should therefore ensure that quality is the focus of attention for all who contribute to our service, that is all our staff.

The strategy will therefore ensure that:

• Patients' needs as individuals are paramount
• Quality is demonstrated by all employees
• The quality aspects of the Trust's purpose and goals are fulfilled
• Patient and customer expectations are identified, met and where possible exceeded
• Value for money is demonstrated
• Value is added to the business of the Trust
• Clinical directors and managers are held accountable for the quality of service for which they are responsible
• The Trust operates a timely and accessible service to all who use it

---

statement that reflects the trust's commitment to a quality service and outlines its overall aims for achieving that service (Box 9.3).

A culture that fosters teamwork in the pursuit of excellence requires a supportive structure that will facilitate its creation. Within an NHS trust, the trust Board is ultimately responsible for the quality of service delivery, and one member of the board is usually identified at all levels within the organisation whose remit is to ensure that the strategic aims identified in the quality strategy are both understood and achieved within their sector. Figure 9.4 represents a quality structure within an NHS hospital trust.

Teamwork used effectively within the pursuit of quality will inevitably have hidden advantages for the trust. It will ensure that:

• A wider range of quality improvements are reviewed
• That skills and abilities of all staff are utilised to the full

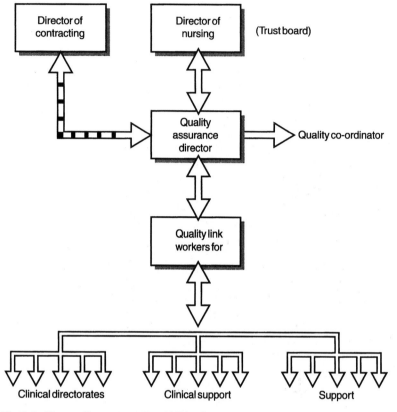

**Fig 9.4**   The quality strategy, Royal Wolverhampton NHS Trust, New Cross Hospital, Wolverhampton

- Job satisfaction and organisational morale are improved because staff are required to be actively involved in improving service quality
- Quality improvements are more readily implemented because of staff involvement in the problem-solving process

---

**Activity 9.3**

Obtain the quality strategy for your own organisation. Familiarise yourself with the strategic aims and objectives.

---

**Activity 9.4**

Draw a diagram of your own organisation's quality structure.

## The scientific approach

The third element of total quality management involves the use of problem-solving methods and data collection techniques that provide accurate statistical feedback which can be used to assure gradual improvement to service quality. Measuring quality involves the setting and monitoring of agreed standards and because of its importance and complexity the measuring of quality will be the main focus of discussion within the remaining sections of this chapter.

## MEASURING QUALITY

### Defining standards and criteria – different approaches

The concept of measurement implies the determination of benchmarks against which something may be compared, e.g. a tape measure used to determine the dimensions of a room. In order for quality to be measured within health care, standards and criteria of achievement need to be established. The task of setting standards is vast, but two models are available to assist this process. The first model, devised by Maxwell (1984), identifies six dimensions that should be addressed by health-care providers in their determination of quality. These dimensions are:

- Accessibility
- Equity
- Relevance to need
- Social acceptability
- Efficiency
- Effectiveness

Box 9.4 describes how these dimensions may be used to formulate standards against which the provision of service within an orthopaedic outpatients department of a NHS hospital trust may be compared.

| Activity 9.5 |
| --- |
| Select an activity which is provided within the department/directorate in which you work and using Maxwell's dimensions write standard statements for your identified activity. |

The second model, devised by Donebedian (1986), has become known as the structure process and outcome model. Donebedian

---

**Box 9.4** Maxwell's dimensions: The provision of an orthopaedic outpatient service

---

**Accessibility – standard**
The Trust should ensure that all patients referred to the Orthopaedic Outpatients Department are offered an appointment within 13 weeks of their referral from the general practitioner and that this access should be as easy as possible.

**Equity – standard**
All patients should receive timely and appropriate orthopaedic outpatient consultation regardless of their race, creed, social class, gender, age and geographical location.

**Relevance to need – standard**
The Trust should offer orthopaedic outpatient consultations which meet the identified needs of patients and purchasers as stipulated in the contracts.

**Social acceptability – standard**
All aspects of the orthopaedic outpatient service must be acceptable to the patients attending the department.

**Efficiency – standard**
The Orthopaedic Outpatient Department service should ensure that consultations are offered, conducted and reported back to the general practitioners without undue delay and at the lowest cost while still ensuring the quality of service.

**Effectiveness – standard**
The Trust should minimise the number of patients who die or suffer undue pain or disability from an orthopaedic condition within its contracted service provision.

**NB** These standards are offered only as examples of the types of standard that may be written using Maxwell's six dimensions as a guide; they do not represent a comprehensive list of standards that should be applied to an outpatient orthopaedic service.

---

advocates that there are three essential areas of consideration when writing standards to assess quality; these are:

- *Structure*, i.e. the physical, financial and organisational resources required to deliver care to the patient
- *Process*, i.e. all the events interactions and interventions that take place during the delivery of care to the patient
- *Outcome*, i.e. The results of care or intervention on the health status of the client or patient

Box 9.5 is an extract from the nursing audit documentation of the Royal Wolverhampton Hospitals NHS Trust and relates to the provision of psychosocial care by the nursing staff. Each standard has been labelled to demonstrate which of the above dimensions it assesses.

---

**Activity 9.6**

Using the same service that you identified in Activity 9.5 and following the example offered in Box 9.5 devise:

- One standard that embraces structure
- One standard that embraces process
- One standard that embraces outcome

---

**Box 9.5** Extract from the nursing audit documentation of an NHS trust demonstrating Donabedian's approach to quality measurement (Royal Wolverhampton NHS Trust Nursing Audit)

*Standard statements for professional nursing: Section A – Psychosocial care*

1. The ward has stated beliefs which are available in the ward philosophy that reflect the psychological needs of the patient. (*Structure*)
2. The nurse conveys interest in the patient. Patient receives full attention from the nurse. Nurse assumes a position which aids communication and observation. (*Process*)
3. The patient is given time to talk. Conversation is encouraged, initiated by the nurse and terminated leaving the patient satisfied. (*Process*)
4. The nurse displays a kind, gentle and friendly but assertive manner. The patient is called by name and is approached with a smile. (*Process*)
5. Expressions of hostility are accepted and changes to care are explained. Withdrawn patients are helped to consider means of involvement. (*Process*)
6. Patient anxiety/distress is noted and appropriate action taken. Questions are posed to ascertain what patient knows about treatment, etc. (*Process*)
7. Patient is helped to explore feelings. Explanation about treatment is provided. Verbal reassurance is given. (*Process*)
8. A full detailed psychosocial assessment is completed within 12 hours. (*Process*)
9. Patients respond positively to the psychosocial interventions employed by the staff. (*Outcome*)

Standard-setting is a time consuming process for most NHS trusts and they have approached the task in a variety of ways. The case study in Box 9.6 describes how the nursing staff of one NHS trust tackled the problem.

**Box 9.6** Case study

The importance of setting and monitoring standards has been recognised within the nursing profession for a number of years and there is a considerable amount of literature available about the mechanics of developing standards however the purpose of this case study is to discuss the process of setting nursing standards within an NHS hospital trust.

The Royal College of Nursing has described a standard as: 'a professionally agreed level of performance appropriate to the population addressed, which is observable, achievable, measurable and desirable' (Royal College of Nursing 1989).

It is vital that the setting of standards locally does not become just another paper exercise, but that the standards are relevant to practice and will result in an improvement in patient care. Our Trust chose to use the dynamic standard setting system (Dyssy), as this was determined to be the most appropriate and advantageous method. This method of developing standards has been used by nurses and other professionals throughout the country in their attempts to set acceptable standards and the system utilises Donabedian's model, which has been described earlier in this chapter, i.e.:

* Structure: What do you need?
* Process: What do you do?
* Outcome: What is the result?

This system was introduced using seminars, workshops, study days and a 'roadshow' that was taken into every ward and department. The aim was to ensure local ownership of the standard-setting process to enable specific operational standards to be developed. It was believed that this would have the possibility of raising the level of care to individual patients. Although standards of excellence are very important, staff have to remain realistic and mindful of available resources. Staff were encouraged to choose topics for standard-setting where nursing input had a significant influence on the outcome for the patient.

Our experience has found that the setting and auditing of standards will only work if the people involved really want it to happen. Setting standards has allowed staff to communicate their standards to others and to participate in peer review, both of which have ensured a higher level of commitment to achievement of quality standards than if they had been imposed from above. Ownership comes with staff creating the standards together and understanding the responsibility they have for their practice.

In recent years professionals within the health service have written standards that apply only to their specific professional role. With greater emphasis being placed on holistic care there is now the need to write standards that embrace a multidisciplinary provision of care. Standard-setting is now being seen as a team effort extending across all disciplines. Corporacy within standard-setting is seen as very important within the Trust while still ensuring the individuality of each speciality.

All members of staff need to be aware of the standards set and the mechanism for peer review, which has proved to be a very effective tool when auditing standards, especially when the practice fails to meet the identified level. Local standards have been found to challenge routine care and facilitate the implementation of research-based practice.

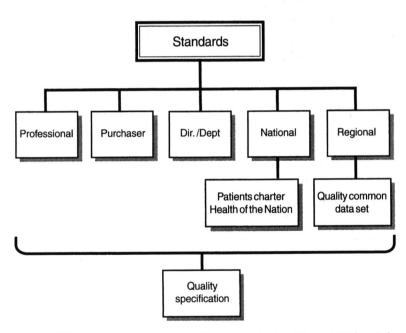

**Fig 9.5** Different perspectives on the setting of standards within an NHS hospital trust

## Setting standards of care – different perspectives
(Fig. 9.5)

Standards within health care are influenced by several factors. These are identified as follows.

## Professional codes of practice

Health-care professionals have established codes of practice that are instigated and disciplined by the professional bodies, e.g. the UKCC Code of Professional Practice for Nurses and Midwives. Standards of care should reflect the requirements of these codes of practice.

## Purchaser requirements

These are stipulated within the contracts that the trust makes with general practitioner fundholders and joint purchasing health authorities (DHAs and FHSAs).

## Directorate/departmental needs

Each trust will have strategic and operational objectives which provide the corporate direction for the organisation. From these the specific quality requirements of the department/directorate will emerge. The type and nature of the service provided by the department or directorate will have an influence on the standards set. Likewise the consumer expectations of that service will also be included and methods identified to assess whether or not such expectations are being met.

## National targets or initiatives

Government initiatives such as the Patient's Charter (Department of Health 1991) and *The Health of the Nation* (Department of Health 1992) identified specific targets and goals for the health service to achieve. These are a very strong influence on the identification of standards within NHS trusts, as there is a requirement on trusts to account for their achievement of these targets.

## Regional directives

The West Midlands region has identified a quality data set, which is a core of information covering a trust's ability to deliver quality services. It has three aims:

1. To rationalise the many and often varied demands for quality information made of providers
2. To provide purchasers with a core of data, in a common format, which they can use to monitor their contracts and inform purchasing decisions
3. To act as an organisational development process which will assist the organisation in achieving its quality improvement objectives (West Midlands Regional Health Authority 1995)

## MONITORING AND REVIEW

The quality cycle or review process is described diagrammatically in Figure 9.6. However, a crucial part of the review process is monitoring of care. There is often confusion between the terms 'monitoring', 'audit' and 'evaluation'. These terms are often used loosely and synonymously, implying that they mean the same thing. It is important therefore to clarify the terms before a more detailed discussion on how quality is monitored is undertaken. Morgan & Everett (1990) offer the following definitions.

**Monitoring**: 'The continuous or regularly repeated observations or measurements of important parts of the service structure process output or outcome'.

**Audit**: 'A discrete activity comprising a detailed periodic review of part or whole of a service or of a procedure. In audit there is an explicit

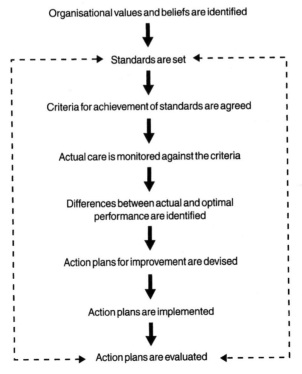

**Fig 9.6** The quality cycle or review process

search for improvement, as with correction: this means that the importance of an audit extends beyond monitoring into service development .

**Evaluation:** 'Refers to the judgements made on information arising from a monitoring system'.

## The monitoring process

Morgan & Everett (1990) identified four stages to the monitoring process:

* Measurement and observation
* Feedback
* Comparison
* Action

This process is explained diagrammatically in Figure 9.7.

A vast amount of data is available to trusts, but auditing tends to be the coordinating thread that draws the information together. Auditing within the NHS until very recently has been uniprofessional, in that each profession (medicine, nursing and the professions allied to medicine – PAM) has developed its own auditing processes. Within the nursing profession various audit tools have been developed, e.g. Monitor, Qualpacs, Slater Nursing Competencies Rating Scale and Phaneuf; however it is very important that audit tools are appropriate to the environment of the audit. It is unlikely that an audit tool that is relevant to the Outpatient Department will suit the needs of the Intensive Care Unit. For that reason nurses have tended to develop

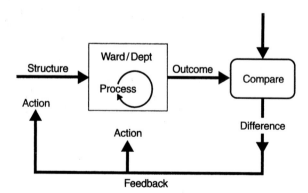

**Fig 9.7** Monitoring quality: a flow chart (Royal Wolverhampton NHS Trust, New Cross Hospital, Wolverhampton)

| Standard | Scores | | | | | | |
|---|---|---|---|---|---|---|---|
| Signs of pain and discomfort are noted and appropriate action is taken | Best Care | Between | Average | Between | Poorest Care | Not Applicable | Not Observed |
| | Score 5 | Score 4 | Score 3 | Score 2 | Score 1 | Score 0 | Score 0 |
| | | | | | | | |

**Fig 9.8** An example of scoring used within the measurement of nursing standards; the scoring key is derived from the Qualpac and Slater quality patient care scales

their own *nursing audit* tools and have identified their own standards and criteria for achievement, which have been locally agreed. Most auditing tools use a system of scoring for quantifying achievement – see Figure 9.8 for an example.

The medical profession has developed its own approach to auditing and four types of *medical audit* have been identified by Ovretveit (1992).

**Internal retrospective audit using peer review:** This is the simplest and most commonly used method of medical audit and involves the retrospective review of the clinical care given to the patient using the patient's records. The audit is internal to a speciality or a hospital and uses a system of peer review to determine areas of clinical practice that could be improved and that would further enhance patient recovery.

**External retrospective audit:** This is a retrospective review of patient care using medical records, but is undertaken in cooperation with other outside groups and can even be a national audit, e.g. *The Confidential Enquiry into Perioperative Deaths* (Buck 1987).

**Concurrent active audit:** This involves conducting a review of patient care while the patient is still receiving care. In concurrent audit the patient's care is usually assessed against agreed protocols or clinical plans.

**Criterion-based audit:** This involves the setting of specific standards of achievement against which actual care can be measured. When specific standards are agreed for identified cases it is possible to compare performance across hospitals.

The emphasis placed by the Government on trusts providing continuity of care for patients, both across disciplines within the hospital and across the hospital and community services, has predisposed the need to move auditing from its uniprofessional approach to a multiprofessional approach. This is referred to as *clinical audit*. Uniprofessional auditing has demonstrated that patients do not usually experience poor quality of care within a single discipline but at the boundaries of care between disciplines. This poor service is not effectively demonstrated by auditing that remains specific to each discipline, so NHS trusts are now emphasising the need for and encouraging a coordinated multidisciplinary approach. One way of achieving this is for staff to become involved in devising collaborative care protocols for patients. These protocols can then identify multidisciplinary standards that can be used in the auditing process.

Within audit much of the data collected is of a qualitative nature, however quantitative data may be collected by the use of *performance indicators*. These are standards that can be determined in numerical or statistical format. Table 9.2 gives an example of how one NHS trust has used statistical data to evaluate its effectiveness in achieving one of the patients' rights identified in the Patient's Charter (Department of Health 1991).

### Stage 1: Measurement and observation
When measuring and reviewing care there are several methods open to NHS trusts – examples include:

- Peer review
- Audit
- Performance indicators
- Individual performance review of staff
- Customer surveys
- Reports from outside bodies, e.g. community health councils
- Complaints

### Stage 2: Feedback
Data collected on audit must be fed back to staff involved. Staff at every level should be involved in the auditing process and aware of the standards achieved. This is imperative if staff are to develop a sense of responsibility for quality and implement improvements as they are agreed.

**Table 9.2** The Royal Wolverhampton Hospitals NHS Trust – Patient's Charter performance (**Charter standard**: Waiting time for treatment in Accident & Emergency; **Standard definition**: No patient will wait longer than 3 hours for treatment after arriving in A & E)

| Hospital | Standard | Total patients treated | 1/10/1994 (%) | Total patients treated | 2/10/1994 (%) | Total patients treated | 3/10/1994 (%) | Total patients treated | 4/10/1994 (%) |
|---|---|---|---|---|---|---|---|---|---|
| Paediatrics – Royal Hospital | (0–5 years) Within 30 minutes | 2694 | 45.53 | 2179 | 60.38 | 2847 | 58.27 | 3111 | 65.43 |
| Adults – Royal Hospital | Within 3 hours | 11 737 | 90.27 | 11 892 | 100 | 15 639 | 92.81 | 15 552 | 94.8 |
| Wolverhampton Eye Infirmary | Treatment within $1\frac{1}{2}$ hours | 11 025 | 82.7 | 11 303 | 89.3 | 10 885 | 84 | 10 320 | 91.4 |

## Stage 3: Comparison

The actual standards of care observed on audit are compared against the previously agreed levels of achievement and differences are noted. These differences may not always be negative where standards observed do not reach those previously agreed, but there may also be areas where actual standards of care exceed the previously agreed standard. In this situation the directorate, ward or department may be noted as having an example of excellent practice that should be shared and noted throughout the trust.

---

**Activity 9.7**

Has your ward or department been audited recently? If so, what areas of good practice were noted? Where did your care fall short of the standard expected?

---

## Stage 4: Action

Auditing should always result in an action plan for improvement. If the audit does not result in changed practice it becomes a worthless exercise. Areas of care that fall short of desired practice should be identified and the appropriate action should be determined to improve that aspect of care. It is important to note that improvement often happens gradually and the essential aspect of auditing is to ensure that the trust is demonstrating a positive trend towards achieving its agreed quality targets and goals.

## Organisational accreditation for quality

Accreditation as an organisation of quality is similar to licensing or registration and involves the organisation being accredited by an accrediting agency. For details of accrediting agencies, see the list at the end of this chapter. Accreditation is both a process and a product. The accrediting agency, e.g. the British Standards Institute, has agreed quality standards that organisations must achieve before receiving a recognised quality award. Accreditation for quality is well established within British industry and the kite-mark of the British Standards Institution is now a well recognised symbol of quality on many products produced within the United Kingdom. The service industries are also now beginning to recognise the value of becoming an accredited institution and the advantages this may bring for their institution in the competitive world of the market place.

## CONCLUSION

The success of a trust in providing the highest possible quality service is dependent on leadership which must be open to new ideas, have the capacity to select the right priorities and have total commitment to the principles and the integrity of the organisation.

The authority and responsibility for the establishment, maintenance, support and evaluation of the effectiveness of quality assurance programmes rest with the trust Board.

Although the specifics for managing the quality assurance programme will vary from trust to trust, the programme should include:

- Clear definition of quality assurance and its goals
- Scope of activities
- Assignment of the authority and responsibility for each specific function
- Methods for reviewing the quality of service provided
- Evaluating mechanisms for reviewing the quality assurance programme
- Methods for communicating the progress with the programme and specific activities

The purpose of any quality assurance programme within a health-care organisation is to maintain existing standards, solve problems that affect patient care and continuously strive to enhance the quality of service provided.

## APPENDIX: ACCREDITING AGENCIES AND ORGANISATIONS THAT WILL PROVIDE FURTHER INFORMATION ON QUALITY ISSUES

British Standards Institution (BSI), Linford Wood, Milton Keynes MK14 6LE

The Institute of Quality Assurance (IQA), PO Box 712, 61 Southwark Street, London SE1 1SB

The European Foundation for Quality Management (EFQM), Avenue des Pleiades, 1200 Brussels, Belgium

The British Quality Foundation (BQF), Vigilant House, 120 Wilton Road, London SW1V 1JZ

National Society for Quality through Teamwork (NSQT), 2 Castle Street, Salisbury, Wiltshire SP11 1BB

Quality Methods Association (QMA), 6a St Mary's Bridge, Plymouth Road, Plympton, Plymouth PL7 4JR

## REFERENCES

Ball J A (1989) Teaching materials quality assurance unit. Nuffield Institute for Health Service Studies, University of Leeds, Leeds

Buck N (1987) Report of a confidential enquiry into postoperative deaths. Nuffield Provincial Hospitals Trust, Kings Fund, London

British Standards, BS5750. British Standards Institute, London

Collard R, Sivyer G, Deloitte L (1990) Total quality. Personnel Management 29 May 1990

Department of Health (1991) The Patient's Charter. HMSO, London

Department of Health (1992) The health of the nation. HMSO, London

Donebedian A (1986) Criteria and standards for quality assessment and monitoring. Quality Rev Bull 2(3): 99–100

Five Regional Consortium (1991) Using information in managing the nursing resource quality. Greenhalgh & Co, Macclesfield

Hill T, Russell M, Gill S, Marchment M (1990) Quality management training manual. Open Software Library, Kall Kwik Printing, St Helens

Joiner B L, Scholtes P R (1985) Total quality leadership v management by control. Joiner & Associates, Sydney, Australia

Maxwell R (1984) Quality assurance in health. Br Med J 12 May: 1470–1472

Maxwell R (1985) Quality assessment in health. In: Management perspectives for doctors. King Edward Hospital Fund for London, p 99

Morgan J, Everett T (1990) In introducing quality management. A training manual. South East Staffordshire Health Authority in conjunction with Birmingham University, Kall Kwik Printing, St Helens

NHS Executive (EL (95) 121) Implementation of new complaints procedure – interim guidelines. NHS Executive, London

Ovretveit J (1992) Health service quality. An introduction to quality methods for health services. Blackwell, Oxford

Royal College of Nursing (1989) Quality patient care. The dynamic standard setting system, Standards of Care Project. Royal College of Nursing, London

West Midlands Regional Health Authority (1995) Sigma quality data set. NHS Executive, Birmingham

# Index

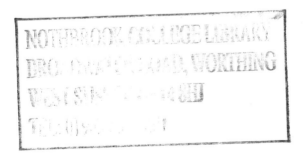